HOSPICE
The Nursing Perspective

Sylvia H. Schraff, MSN, RN
Coordinating Editor

Pub. No. 20-1967

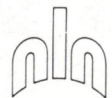

National League for Nursing • New York

Copyright © 1984 by
National League for Nursing

ISBN 0-88737-119-1

All rights reserved. No part of this book may be reproduced in print, or by photostatic means, or in any other manner, without the express written permission of the publisher.

Manufactured in the United States of America

Contents

INTRODUCTION *ix*
  Sylvia H. Schraff

ABOUT THE AUTHORS *xiii*

1 WHAT MAKES HOSPICE UNIQUE? *1*
  Rachel E. Spector
Historical Review *2*
  Antecedents of Hospital and Hospice *3*
  Modern Day Hospital and Hospice *3*
Philosophical Underpinnings *4*
  Curing Philosophies *4*
  Healing Philosophies *6*
  Palliative Care *7*
  Comprehensive Approach to Care *9*
  Amount of Care *10*
Providers' Basic Beliefs *11*
Summary *13*
Notes *13*
References *14*

308716

2 ORGANIZATION AND ADMINISTRATION 17
Mary Lou Gillespie and Karen Freeman Gartland

Emphasis on Home Care 18
Community Involvement 19
Hospice Development 20
    Gaining Community Support 20
    Assessing Community Needs and Resources 20
    Organizational Models 22
Organizational Structures 25
    Medicare Reimbursement 26
    Size of Agency 27
Financing the Hospice 27
Administrative Structures 28
    Contracting 32
    Marketing 32
Summary 33
Notes 34
References 34

3 REIMBURSEMENT ISSUES 35
S. Jill Schultz

The Medicare Regulations—TEFRA 1982 38
    Rules and Regulations 38
    Reimbursement 40
    Issues 40
Conclusions 45
Notes 45
References 46

4 THE HOSPICE TEAM 47
Myra J. Downs

The Team Concept 47
    Qualifications of Team Members 48
Team Coordination 48
    Team Support Group 49
    Record Keeping 51
Role of the Nurse 51

Roles of Other Team Members 53
    Chaplain 53
    Medical Social Worker 53
    Speech/Language Pathologist 53
    Dentist 54
    Nutritionist 54
    Occupational Therapist 55
    Physical Therapist 55
    Pharmacist 55
    Home Health Aide 56
    Psychologist 56
    Medical Director 56
Summary 57
Notes 57
References 57
Sample Job Descriptions 58

5 STAFFING AND STRESS MANAGEMENT 73
Barbara M. Petrosino

Criteria for Staff Selection 73
    Motivation 74
    Other Characteristics 74
Applications and Interviews 75
Orientation 77
Staffing Needs 79
Scheduling 81
    Inpatient Units 81
    Home-Care Programs 81
    On-Call Assignments 81
Sources of Stress 82
    Hospice Care as a Stressor 82
    Organizational Sources of Stress 84
    Personal Characteristics 85
Indicators of Stress 86
Strategies for Managing Stress 86
    Personal Actions 87
    Support Services 88

Personnel Polices 89
Opportunities for Professional Growth 89
Notes 90
References 91

6 THE ROLE OF THE NURSE 93
Barbara M. Petrosino and Marlene H. Weitzel

The Nurse as Administrator 93
    Community Relations 93
    Quality Assurance 94
The Nurse as Caregiver 95
    The Family 95
    The Nursing Process in Hospice Care 97
    Death in the Home 102
Ethical Decision Making 106
    Patient Situation 107
Notes 111
References 113

7 VOLUNTEERS 117
Diane S. Pedersen

Introduction 117
Organization and Financial Issues 118
    Conflict of Philosophies 118
    Funding 119
Roles and Responsibilities 119
Recruitment and Screening 121
    The Screening Process 122
Training and Evaluation 123
    Training Programs 123
    A Competency-Based Approach 125
    Evaluation Methods 126
Coordination of Volunteers 128
Notes 129
References 129

8 HOSPICE BEREAVEMENT PROGRAMS: TRENDS AND ISSUES 131
Alice S. Demi

Philosophy of Bereavement Care 131
    Crisis Theory 132
    Bereavement Adaptation 132
    Concurrent Crises 132
    Need for Bereavement Services 134
    Anticipatory Grief 134
    Goals of Bereavement Programs 135
    Assessing Client Progress 136
    Evaluating Bereavement Services 137
Types of Services 137
    Preparation for Bereavement 139
    Funeral Visits 139
    Home Visits and Telephone Follow-Up 139
    Educational Programs 140
    Memorial Services 140
    Social Groups 140
    Self-Help and Support Groups 140
    Comprehensive Bereavement Services 141
The Bereavement Team 141
    Model Training Curriculum 142
Standards for Bereavement Services 143
Concerns and Issues 145
Summary 146
Notes 147
References 149

9 CURRENT ISSUES AND FUTURE DIRECTIONS 153
Jessie F. Igou

Nature and Scope of Practice with Hospice Patients 153
    Physiological Dimension 154
    Emotional Dimension 156
    Spiritual Dimension 158
Nature and Scope of Practice with Hospice Families 160
Meeting the Needs of Hospice Staff 163

Research *164*
    Clinical Effectiveness *164*
    Cost Effectiveness *164*
Summary *165*
Notes *165*
References *167*

CASE EXAMPLES
Home-Health-Agency-Based Hospice *169*
A Community-Based Hospice *183*
Merger: Hospice and VNA *191*
Hospice Care, Inc.—A For-Profit Company *199*
Hospital-Based Hospice *203*
Long-Term-Care-Facility-Based Hospice Program *217*

Introduction
Sylvia H. Schraff

Hospice: The Nursing Perspective focuses on the uniqueness of hospice and the hospice movement. Nurses have been providing care and comfort to the dying throughout the history of the profession. Nurses have always been with the dying to ease the suffering, share the pain, and make the journey less difficult. They are there in the middle of the night to provide the last human contact to those who are departing this known world. Nurses provide comfort after the news is broken about the inevitability of death. The dying and their loved ones have always made use of the counsel of nurses to help them in difficult situations. For all these reasons, hospice is a natural for nurses. This book attempts to give the reader a view of the hospice movement from the angle of nursing and to point out the importance of the role of nursing in this movement.

When I was asked to edit this proposed volume on hospice, I accepted only on the condition that the text would not only come from a nursing focus but that a clear distinction would be made between hospice and traditional care. From my perspective as a community health nurse and a director of a community home health and hospice organization, I felt that the differences had not been covered adequately. The hospice movement gained popularity across the nation shortly after it was introduced. Everyone seemed to want to get on the bandwagon; hospices sprang up everywhere. Some focused on the psychological and spiritual aspects of dying, others on physical care, while some gave traditional care but under a new name. Some hospices appeared to focus on the needs of the terminally ill, but some, unfortunately, exploited the dying in favor of their own vested interests. Doctors, nurses, clergy, social workers, therapists, counselors, and many other professionals competed to carve out their niches in this new movement. Now that the initial surge has passed, it is time to go back to the basics and explore the uniqueness of the hospice concept as well as the contributions that nursing and other disciplines can make in the effort to promote healthy dying.

Dying is as much a part of living as is birthing, but the naturalness of death has been denied and the subject has been avoided, especially in this past century. Death was often felt to be a failure, an inability to control life's forces, a defeat in the battle to survive. The hospice movement has helped us focus on dying as part of living, and healthy living as well as dying is becoming accepted as a goal in itself.

Hospice encompasses concepts of healthy dying and healthy grieving. Rabbi Abraham Hershel explains that "death may be the beginning of exaltation, an unlimited celebration, a reunion of the divine source of being." He continues that, with death, "the image, the divine stake in man, is restored to the bundle of life. Death is not sensed as a defeat, but as a summation, a conclusion."

Healthy dying also encompasses the right of choice about one's own care. Mutuality in goal setting is an important aspect of hospice care. Team members work closely with the patient and the family to provide care that is acceptable to all involved. Martha Rogers states that "goal setting encompasses both preservation and enhancement of meaningful life and a meaningful transition from life to death" (*Theoretical Basis of Nursing*, F.A. Davis, 1970, p. 125). For death to be meaningful, hospice workers must secure what has relevance and is important to their patients.

Almost all of the terminally ill patients I have known have chosen to die at home. The authors of *Home Care: Living with Dying* state that "home is truly a person's castle. There one is master. Within one's home, humble though it may be, one has the security of being surrounded by familiar objects—objects that have meaning and value to oneself alone. They stir memories. Only in one's home does one have the freedom to eat what one desires, when one desires it. Only here does one have the freedom to bathe, dress and sleep when one wishes" (Columbia University Press, 1979, p. 5). The importance of dying at home seems to be coupled with the need for freedom and the need for preserving choice.

Healthy grieving is as important as healthy dying in the hospice philosophy. Grieving is a natural process that eventually can lead to remembrance of pleasant experiences and happy moments or can deteriorate into obsessive self-reproach and guilt over past problems. The hospice caregiver is important in helping people use the powerful forces within them during this time and in helping them move on to new experiences and new memories in a healthy fashion.

Hospice: The Nursing Perspective is intended not only for members of the nursing profession but also for members of other disciplines. Because care of the dying transcends any one professional discipline, various professionals may find all or portions of the book valuable. Direct-service providers, such as those comprising the interdisciplinary team, as well as instructors, students, and interested lay people can find materials here that will give them a broader base of understanding of the concept of hospice and perhaps convince them of the importance of ensuring that dying people have access to the advantages of such a program.

The text is divided into two parts. The first is composed of chapters on selective topics on hospice as a concept, the organization and administration of hospice programs, the components of the program, the roles of the team members, as well as issues and future directions. The second half, starting on page 169, moves from the conceptual level to real-life examples of the development of hospice programs in a variety of settings.

Chapter 1 is a beautiful essay entitled "What Makes Hospice Unique?" This first chapter provides an overview of the philosophical underpinnings of the curing, healing, and palliative care concepts and outlines for the reader a comprehensive approach to care of the dying. Chapter 2 is a detailed description of the organization of a hospice program, the structure of administrative lines of authority, and the establishment of relationships within the community. Reimbursement issues are dealt with in Chapter 3, which also discusses the future needs of hospice programs. Chapter 4 is devoted to the concept of the team and the role of the team members. A highlight of this chapter is a section on coordination of care.

Chapter 5 is a comprehensive discussion of selecting staff members for the hospice program and helping them deal with the stresses associated with working exclusively with the dying. Chapter 6 outlines the role of the nurse as an administrator and as a caregiver in hospice, applies the nursing process to care of the terminally ill, and provides examples of the use of nursing diagnosis.

The role of volunteers in the hospice program is covered in Chapter 7. Steps in recruitment, screening, and training are discussed, as well as ways to ensure success of this key component of the hospice program. Chapter 8 outlines the philosophical issues of bereavement, types of bereavement services, and the role of the team. An interesting section on a survey of hospice bereavement programs can provide the reader with a better understanding of the perceived strengths as well as limitations of these programs. The last chapter explores the current issues that face hospice programs and clarifies those issues to provide direction for the future.

The six Case Examples that follow depict the actual development of hospices in existing organizations such as hospitals, home health agencies, and nursing homes, as well as freestanding hospice programs and a description of a merger between a freestanding hospice and a VNA. These first-hand descriptions of the actual development of hospice programs include not only the successes but also the problems encountered on the way. It is hoped that the reader will benefit from this sharing of experiences and be stimulated to continue the quest for better ways to serve the dying.

As an editor of a multiauthored text, one has many accolades to pass out. I am indebted to the authors, who have most generously taken the time to put on paper their thoughts and insights, their ideas and experiences. These people were selected for their wisdom and their expertise. I am most grateful to them.

I am especially grateful for the help of NLN's staff, especially Elaine Silverstein, without whose guidance and direction this project could not have been undertaken. Also, I would be remiss if I did not mention the staff of the Home Nursing Agency, who not only assisted me with data collections, typing, and other such tasks, but gave me their support and encouragement.

I trust that this book will help nurses and others involved in providing hospice services gain insight and information that will help them find ways to better help the dying. I also hope that the concept of healthy dying is contagious and that practitioners "catch" the urge to become more competent and effective in caring for the dying person, for in the course of time, we all will need such compassionate care.

About the Authors

Sister Dolores Castellano, MS, RN, a member of the Congregation of the Infant Jesus, is the founder and director of the Hospice Program at Mercy Hospital, Rockville Centre, Long Island, New York. A member of the board of directors of the New York State Hospice Association, Sister has given many lectures on hospice and has served as consultant to colleagues seeking to establish hospice programs.

Alice S. Demi, DNSc, RN, FAAN, is professor and chairperson, Department of Community Health Nursing, School of Nursing, Medical College of Georgia, Augusta. Dr. Demi was formerly the coordinator of nursing services at the Hospice of Marin and a director of the Hospice of Metropolitan Denver. She has spoken and published widely on hospice and conducted research on the outcomes of bereavement.

Myra J. Downs, MSN, RN, is currently a consultant for the development of the Etowah County Hospice Organization in Alabama and serves as secretary to the hospice advisory board. In the past, she has developed both hospital- and community-based hospice programs and has published several articles on hospice and spoken on the subject throughout the Southeast.

Karen Freeman Gartland, MS, RN, is team director for Dallas Hospice Care, Inc. Before assuming this position in January 1984, she was director of nursing therapy for the Visiting Nurse Association of Dallas Home Hospice Program. She is an active member of the American and Texas Nurses' Associations, the Texas and American Public Health Associations, and the Texas Hospice Organization.

Mary Lou Gillespie, MPH, RN, is currently the executive director of Dallas Hospice Care, Inc. She is active in the National and Texas Hospice Organizations, the American and Texas Nurses' Associations, the Texas Public Health Association, and both national and state hospice councils. She has spent 25 years in community health service, 18 of which have been in an administrative or supervisory capacity. She has given numerous presentations, both regionally and nationally.

Jessie Igou, DrPH, RN, is assistant professor of nursing at The Pennsylvania State University with responsibility for teaching graduate and undergraduate courses in gerontology, community health, and concepts of health. Dr. Igou's previous experience was in long-term care, both in inpatient institutions and home health agencies. She has developed and implemented continuing education programs on care of the dying patient and family and served on a hospice board of directors.

Sister Karen McNally, MSA, RN, is a member of The Sisters of Mercy, Province of Baltimore. Sister is associate administrator of the Cardinal Shehan Center for the Aging, Towson, Maryland, and has previously served as a staff nurse both in Guyana and the United States and as a director of nursing service. She is a member of the Home Health Care Professional Advisory Committee, Mercy Hospital, Baltimore, Maryland; of the Home Health Care Professional Advisory Committee, Saint Agnes Hospital, Baltimore, Maryland; and of the board of directors, Health Facilities Association of Maryland.

Diane Pedersen, MPH, RN, CNP, is director, Home Care/Hospice, St. Agnes Hospital, Baltimore, Maryland, and president of the Maryland Association of Home Health Agencies. Formerly a community and school health nurse and adult nurse practitioner, Ms. Pedersen is active in supporting and presenting legislative testimony in support of home health legislation.

Barbara M. Petrosino, EdD, RN, assistant professor of nursing, the University of Texas at Austin, has been active in hospice work for the past six years. She initiated and serves as editor of the *Hospice Nursing Newsletter,* which currently is distributed to 2,000 nurses nationwide. She has participated in nearly every capacity in the development of Hospice of El Paso and has most recently served as its president. Among other activities, she has conducted workshops on death and dying, currently serves as chairperson of the professional liaison committee of the National Hospice Organization, and is an associate editor for nursing of *The Hospice Journal,* a new publication scheduled for distribution in early 1985.

Sylvia H. Schraff, MSN, RN, is executive director of the Home Nursing Agency of Blair, Huntingdon, and Fulton Counties, Altoona, Pennsylvania, and instructor in community health nursing at Saint Francis College, Loretto, Pennsylvania. Ms. Schraff is active in many public health and professional organizations and is chairperson of the executive committee, Gerontological Nursing Division, American Nurses' Association, and chairperson of the executive committee of the Council on Community Health Services, National League for Nursing.

S. Jill Schultz, MS, RN, executive director of the VNA of Saginaw, Saginaw, Michigan, has held a variety of positions in health care organizations, both hospitals and home health agencies. She has been associated with the VNA of Saginaw for the last nine years, and has been executive director since 1980. She is active in the NLN/APHA accreditation program for community health agencies and has been listed in *Who's Who* among American women in finance and industry.

Rachel E. Spector, PhD, RN, is currently associate professor, Boston College School of Nursing, teaching community health and oncology nursing and cultural diversity in health and illness. Dr. Spector has published and lectured widely on cultural factors in health and illness and is the author of *Cultural Diversity in Health and Illness*.

Marlene H. Weitzel, PhD, RN, is assistant dean, College of Nursing and Allied Health, the University of Texas at El Paso. Dr. Weitzel has held various faculty and administrative positions in nursing education programs in Texas, Arizona, New York, South Dakota, and Nebraska. She has been a coauthor of a well-received fundamentals of nursing textbook for the past four editions and is interested in nursing ethics, nursing process, and nursing theory development.

Chapter 1
What Makes Hospice Unique?
Rachel E. Spector

I recall meeting a colleague in a Boston park ten years ago. It was a misty, cold March afternoon, but we decided to meet on a deserted park bench rather than in a more public location. No, we were neither spies nor drug dealers—we were meeting against the advice of the director of the agency where I was employed, and we preferred not to be seen together. The purpose of our meeting was to discuss strategies for introducing a hospice to the greater Boston area. Each of us had collected anecdotal data to demonstrate the need for such a facility; each of us was committed to this goal.

What nurse who has been practicing for even one or two years has not witnessed the resuscitation of a terminally ill cancer patient? Who cannot remember the hopeless cries of both young and elderly patients who have been left alone to die? The silent or not-so-silent anguish of families? The frustration of performing needless, costly, and painful procedures on unwilling patients? The anguish of family members who are left to wait outside the ICU doors? The feelings of empty frustration?

All of us have ghosts in our closets of memories. We all remember those special patients whom we could not help, whose pain defied alleviation, whose family could not be comforted, either because we were too busy with "life-saving" work or because we did not know what to say.

Imagine a barren tree trunk—alone, isolated, deserted, withered, bleak, dark, threatening—something to fear and run from. Slowly, over the course of time, a few little twigs begin to sprout from the trunk of this lonely tree. Then, as time passes, the twigs bud and blossoms appear. There is yet a glimmer of hope.

The analogy is to death, the attitudes and conditions surrounding an event that we as humans all share. The barren trunk is the frame of reference we implanted in our nursing students in the past. I remember as a student being taught to "tag the big toe and insert dentures" and not much more, when care of the dying was the class topic. There were no discussions about the meaning of life and death, the experiences and concerns of the patient and family, and the feelings the nurse might have. If someone could not cope with the all-too-numerous deaths in the hospital setting, she was advised to leave nursing; the profession was not for her. As technology improved throughout the 1950s, 1960s, and 1970s, this attitude became more ingrained. When a patient died it was due to "neglect" on the part of the physician and nurse, and all too often we became liable for the death. Surely, with all the life-saving means available through technology, no one should or could die. This attitude reached its peak in the late '70s, when nearly every death became a "code." Patients did not die—they "coded."

Slowly, some changes in attitude began to occur. In 1972, I attended a lecture by Dr. Elisabeth Kubler-Ross. She actually talked about death. She broke taboos. She forced me, and the rest of the audience, to think and to confront troubling emotions. She and several others forced the barren tree trunk to begin to sprout.

Shortly thereafter the concept of hospice began to encroach on the consciousness of nurses and other health care professionals. The buds . . . a ray of hope, change from the painful, dehumanized care we were all forced to provide for patients. Hospice offered an alternative, a different philosophy, a different approach to terminal care. It provided a feeling of hope, substance, caring, and humaneness, where before there was depersonalization, dehumanization, and despair.

The hospice movement has exploded during the past ten years. At the present time (1984) there are at least 1,500 hospices in the United States, and interest in the movement continues to swell. The purpose of this chapter is to describe the unique nature of hospice care.

The question "what makes hospice unique?" can be answered by: (1) comparing the history and philosophy of the hospital and the hospice and (2) analyzing philosophies of curing and healing.

HISTORICAL REVIEW

It is not within the scope of this chapter to present an indepth discussion of the history of the hospital and hospice movements; however, a brief comparison of the concepts and their development is warranted.

Antecedents of Hospital and Hospice

Both *hospital* and *hospice* are derived from the Latin word *hospes*—a guest, a host.[1] The noun *hospital* is further derived from the Latin *hospitale*—a house, inn; *hospice* from the Latin *hospitium,* hospitality, an inn, lodging. Both words share a common root, yet they have evolved separately.

Hospital is defined today as an institution where the ill or injured may receive medical, surgical, or psychiatric treatment, nursing, food and lodging, etc., during illness. *Hospice* has two definitions: (1) a place of refuge for travelers, especially that belonging to the monks of Saint Bernard in the Alps; (2) a home for the sick or poor. (Both definitions come from *Webster's New Twentieth Century Dictionary, Unabridged.*)

Hospitals. Hospitals developed over the millennia out of a sense of humanitarianism and brotherhood. The first era in the development of hospitals was over four thousand years ago, when priests performed rites to cure sickness. In Eygpt and ancient Babylon, illness was treated by priest-physicians. Twenty-five hundred years ago the Greeks developed health temples, and the practices employed within the temples gave evidence of a sophisticated knowledge and understanding of the body and mind. Christians developed the ideal of giving loving care and compassion to the poor, the sick, outcasts, and the dying, and hospitals began to develop.[2] The hospital as we know it today has evolved into a giant megastructure with goals that differ greatly from providing loving, compassionate care. The shortcomings of the modern hospital—its emphasis on efficiency, on technology, on hierarchical structure, on curing the patient at all costs—have led to the development of the hospice.

Hospice. A *hospice,* as the word is used in this book, is a medically directed multidisciplinary program providing skilled care of an appropriate nature for terminally ill patients and their families, thus allowing the patients to live as fully as possible until death. Hospice helps relieve symptoms of the distress (physical, psychological, spiritual, social, economic) that may occur during the course of the disease, dying, and bereavement.[3] Hospice is further described as a program of care in which an organized interdisciplinary team systematically provides palliative care (medical relief of pain) and supportive services to dying patients.[4]

Modern Day Hospital and Hospice

Just as one can see the changes in the meanings of the terms hospital and hospice, so too has change occurred in the services provided by each institution. As caregivers within hospitals grew more and more skilled in technological care, they became less and less able to comfort and care for the terminally ill. The demand for humane care arose, and hospice was the response to this demand. The revitalization of hospices as places for the care of the dying after several centuries of disuse is credited to Dr. Cicely Saunders in England and Dr. Elisabeth Kubler-Ross in the United States.

The ancient term *hospice* was first revived in England by the Irish Sisters of Charity, who opened homes for the dying during the nineteenth century. Dr. Cicely Saunders, who in the late 1940s lost a friend to cancer, shared a dream with this friend: to create a quiet place where people could die with peace and dignity. The man endowed Dr. Saunders with funds to establish a place like the nineteenth-century hospice, and St. Christopher's Hospice, London, was born.[5]

Early in the 1960s Dr. Saunders visited the Yale–New Haven Hospital in New Haven, Connecticut, and eloquently described St. Christopher's Hospice and the needs of the dying. After a long and arduous struggle, funds were raised to begin a hospice, and in 1974 patients in the New Haven area began to receive home care. The National Cancer Institute and the Kaiser Foundation provided start-up funding for the fledgling program. By 1976 New Haven was receptive to the hospice concept and the movement rooted and sprouted.[6]

PHILOSOPHICAL UNDERPINNINGS

Hospice care is a humane, sensible approach to terminal illness, for it is designed to provide care, comfort, and support of family and friends as death approaches. This caring philosophy is a marked departure from the underlying philosophy of hospital care in that it does not concern itself with curing the disease but with healing the patient. A holistic approach is taken to patient and family care.

Curing Philosophies

The differences between hospital care and hospice care for the terminally ill are most dramatically apparent when one analyzes the philosophical underpinnings of these two institutions. The philosophy of the modern hospital is to prevent death, literally at all costs to the patient and the family; the hospice philosophy is to help the patient and the family acknowledge and deal with the realities of impending death and to prepare themselves physically, mentally, and spiritually for the event.

> Whereas the hospital expects to discharge 97.5 percent of its patients, the hospice expects to remain with its patients until they die.

TABLE 1.1
COMPARISON: HOSPITAL AND HOSPICE CARE

	Hospital	Hospice
Problem	Acute illness	Terminal illness
Outcome	Discharge (97.5%)	Death
Setting	Institutional	Home with institutional backup
Environment	Sterile	Home
Type of care	Curative	Comfort
Caregivers	Hierarchy	Team
Length of stay	7.3 days (average)	6 months
Family involvement	Peripheral	Extensive involvement

Source: Adapted from Susan Burger, "Three Approaches to Patient Care: Hospice, Nursing Homes, and Hospitals," in Michael Hamilton and Helen Reid, eds., *A Hospice Handbook: A New Way to Care for the Dying* (Grand Rapids, Mich.: William B. Eerdman, 1980), p. 132.

Whereas the hospital setting is impersonal, noisy, cold, dark, and sterile, hospice care is often given in the patient's home or in an institution that has been designed to be homelike and peaceful.

Whereas hospital care is designed by the nature of the institution to be curative, hospice care is designed to be palliative and healing and to provide comfort to the patient and family.

Whereas hospital care is given by caregivers bound by custom to a hierarchy of control and command, hospice care is team in nature, with various people in various roles serving as the team leader. For example, the person closest to the patient and the family, often a nurse or social worker, leads and coordinates the care plans.

Whereas the patient's length of stay in the hospital tends to be seven or eight days, a person may be followed by the hospice for six months or longer.

Whereas in the hospital setting the family members are passive and have little or no say in the patient's care, in the hospice they are active. In the hospital the family members are the visitors, the folks who call in, the ones who sit, worry, and wait. All too often they are uninformed and do not understand what is happening; they do not understand medical jargon or know what questions to ask. In the hospice, the family members actively participate in the patient's care. They tell the providers what needs to be done. They orchestrate. They request. They respond. Family members are recognized as a part of the team, and their needs are important and valued as highly as those of the patient.[7]

Healing Philosophies

Healing is an essential concept underlying the hospice philosophy of caring. The word *healing* has deep and complex meaning that can be analyzed in a number of dimensions:

1. **The physical dimension:** A restoration to wholeness. For example, when a lesion, wound, or fracture heals; when a damaged cell regenerates.
2. **The mental dimension.** When one experiences a loss or other emotional stress, the mind, over time, heals.
3. **The spiritual dimension.** When the spirit, which has suffered disease in the form of guilt, sin, or loss of faith, is healed and restored to wholeness either by religious experience or other forms of spiritual awakening and restoration.

Within the context of religious uses of healing, one sees strong emphasis on faith in God. Reference to the healing powers of God are made in the Old and New Testaments and in both Jewish and Christian prayers. The belief that healing is done through Jesus is prevalent among religious Christians. Types of religious healing include:

1. **Spiritual healing** through repentance of sin.
2. **Inner healing** through healing of the memory.
3. **Physical healing** through laying on of hands or speaking in tongues.
4. **Deliverance, or exorcism,** through the deliverance of the sufferer or exorcism of evil.[8]
5. **The holistic dimension:** When one aspect of a person—body, mind, or spirit—is diseased, the problem affects the whole person. In order for the problem to be resolved and for health to be restored, the whole person, body, mind, and spirit, must be healed.

6. **The psychosomatic dimension:** When one's mind is seen as the cause of the physical problem, such as asthma or colitis, the healing approach is to heal the mind in concert with the body.

In the hospice, caring includes a spiritual healing that supports the patient and, of equal importance, supports the survivors and provides a mechanism for healing the wound of death in the loved ones.

Palliative Care

Palliative care is care that aims to alleviate symptoms and to control pain. The control of pain is of primary importance, for it frees patients from deep suffering and helps them to have more time and energy to respond to family and friends and to put their lives in order before dying. Unlike acute care, which is curative in intent, palliative care is designed to sustain the body, mind, and spirit of the dying person.[9]

Pain is the most critical symptom to control in the care of the terminally ill. This pain is not only physical but also social, psychological, and spiritual. Therefore, hospice care is directed not only to the management of physical pain but to the three other types as well.

In dealing with social pain, hospice attempts to help patients live fully until they die, recognizing that patients need someone to talk to, someone to whom they can express feelings of loneliness and anguish. Social pain may manifest itself in one of two ways: (1) the patient's mild-to-severe discomfort with man's inhumanity to man, and (2) changes in interpersonal relationships caused by the patient's learning how to say goodbye. Psychological pain is seen in the frightened or anxious patient—lonely, depressed, hurt, angry. Hospice caregivers give the patient an opportunity to express fears and anger, and often the pain is relieved.

Spiritual pain is undefinable. Yet much of the communication between the dying patient and the caregiver is at a spiritual level. It is in caring for the dying that caregivers begin to sense their own mortality and life. The spiritual needs of patients and their families vary from patient to patient and are predicated on the patient's ethnic, cultural, and religious background.[10] Research indicates that there are differences both within and between ethnoreligious groups regarding individuals' needs and desires for spiritual care. For example, a preliminary study I conducted found a wide variation in the beliefs cancer patients held with respect to their diagnoses and prognoses. Patients with strong ties to their ethnoreligious heritage identified less need for support from networks outside their families and churches, whereas patients who were less tied to their ethnoreligious heritage sought more secular support. Further research is needed in this area before any valid conclusions can be drawn.

Religious teachings offer many answers to questions about life and death, the meaning of life and death, and the meaning of suffering. To some patients and their families these answers provide comfort and relief; to others these answers are either inadequate or unwanted.

Physical pain, be it acute or chronic, may be the most debilitating of the four kinds of pain. It is visible and the symptoms are observable and measurable. The management of physical pain is seen as the key to good hospice care, for when this pain is managed satisfactorily, other symptoms can be controlled. Often the physical pain is protopathic—constant, persistent, and increasing rather than decreasing. Hospice programs include several options for controlling this pain, such as the use of drugs and narcotics (see Chapter 6). There is no maximum dose of pain medication for dying patients, and addiction ought not be a concern.[11]

There are numerous paths leading to the employment of palliative rather than curative care. Figure 1.1 illustrates these paths. In general,

Figure 1.1 Schema of Palliative Care

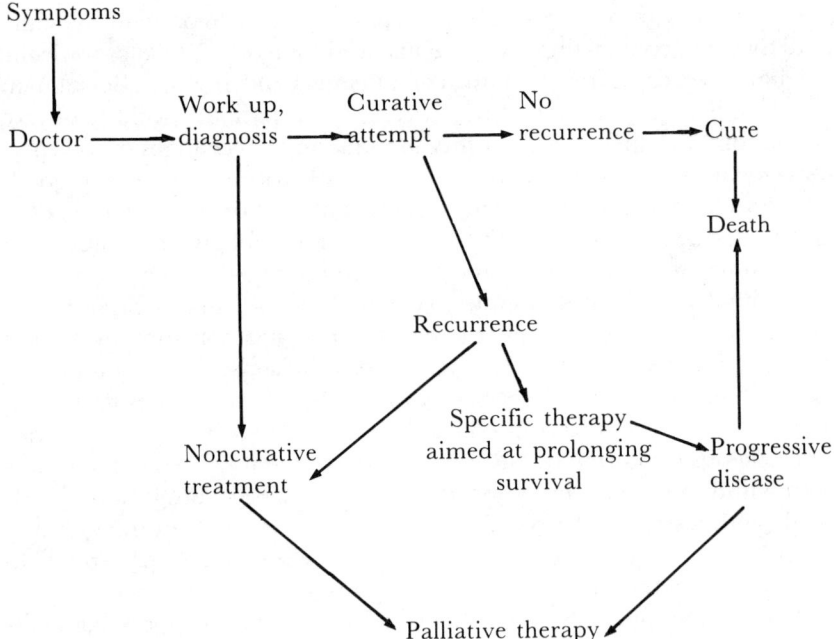

Source: United States Department of Health and Human Services, *Hospice Education Program for Nurses, Modules I-II*. DHHS Publication No. HRA 81-27, June 1981, p. 17.

the patient visits the doctor with symptoms. He is worked up and a diagnosis is determined. Curative care is attempted, and the patient is either cured or not cured. With curing, he may not be seen by the doctor again, or he may develop a recurrence. If treatment is noncurative or disease recurs, the patient will receive either specific therapy to prolong survival or palliative therapy. In either case, disease will progress and ultimately will lead to death. At some point, a choice must be made between continuing various forms of treatment, or searching for ways to provide comfort or palliation. Many people are now selecting palliation.

The philosophy of hospice workers toward the relief of symptoms differs greatly from that of other health care workers, as palliation, the relief of symptoms, is a major focus of treatment in the hospice care.

Comprehensive Approach to Care

The care that the hospice provides is comprehensive and falls into five major categories:

1. **Physiological:** The control of physiological needs are predicated upon the following:
    a. **Adequate communication:** The patient is free to describe symptoms, and all members of the team must be sensitive and alert to symptoms.
    b. **Follow up:** The treatment that is provided must be continually adapted to meet the patient's changing needs.

Included in the physical needs of hospice patients are problems of pain, weakness, thirst, hypercalcemia, hemorrhage, anorexia, dysgeneusia, dysphagia, nausea and vomiting, constipation, diarrhea, intestinal obstruction, ascites, cough, dyspnea, congestion, hiccups, urinary tract infection, incontinence, depression, insomnia, dementia, paralysis, decubitus ulcers, pruritus, and fistulae.[12] The physical problems can occur in any number and in any order. Most can be treated at home and do not require acute-care admissions.

2. **Psychological:** Psychological needs include loneliness and depression. The problems include poor communication with friends and family members. It is often the concerned hospice worker who listens well, who demonstrates caring in both verbal and nonverbal ways, and who is aware of the person and the problem who is most important at this time. The worker listens empathetically and is able to bridge communication gaps between friends and family members. Care is supportive and sensitive.

3. **Sociological:** Hospice patients have many social needs, such as a need for costly supplies. Other needs include transportation and assistance with daily activities and decision making. Problems caused by changes in role and responsibility, in body image and mobility, in work and social relationships must be addressed. The termination of social relationships is often eased with the help of a hospice worker.

4. **Educational.** A wide range of educational needs may develop over the course of hospice care. The patient and family members must be taught how to care for the many physical problems that develop, how to administer medications for pain, and how to prepare food that is palatable and digestible. They must also be taught the significance of each physical problem. Education is ongoing and must be molded to fit the patient's and family's needs.

5. **Spiritual.** For most people facing inevitable death the spiritual problems may well be the most perplexing. What is the meaning of all this? Why me? Even with the time involved in a long illness, as the end approaches the patient will still ask these questions.[13]

Amount of Care

The following care principles are described by Buckingham as appropriate for the care of the dying and their families:

1. The patient needs to be as symptom free as possible so that his energy can be used to live the remaining portion of his life as fully as possible. Any problems that develop on a day-to-day basis must be addressed by the appropriate provider, but unusual means need not be employed.

2. Doctors and nurses must be easily accessible to the patient and to the family.

3. Continuity of care should be maintained, whether the patient is at home or in the hospital.

4. The patient's and the family's life-style must be maintained and their life philosophies respected by the professional health caregivers.

5. Loneliness, isolation, and fear of abandonment are significant sources of concern for dying patients. Professional and lay caregivers must be prepared to address these issues.

6. Twenty-four-hour-a-day care must be available to the patient and the family.
7. No one person can fully meet the needs of the dying. A multidisciplinary team must be available for support, counseling, and advice. This team may include a doctor, a nurse, a social worker, a clergyman, and a lawyer.
8. The patient should be treated as a person, not as a disease, by professional caregivers, family, and friends.
9. Humanistic care should be integrated with expert medical and nursing care.
10. A family that is facing an impending death needs support and advice from health care professionals.
11. The terminal patient must be allowed to give as well as to receive.
12. All caregivers should convey to the dying patient a sense of continuing self-respect and identity as a person with freedom from being a burden to others.
13. The family must feel a sense of participation in decision making.
14. The primary caregiver tending to a patient at home needs support and occasional relief from his or her duties.

PROVIDERS' BASIC BELIEFS

The basic beliefs of those who provide care in the hospice setting differ greatly from those of hospital workers. As has been stated, the hospital's mission is to cure, the hospice's, to care. Therefore, the hospital worker thinks in ways designed to bring about cure; the hospice worker does not. The hospice concept has four basic principles:[14]

1. The patient and the family are the unit of care. The family is essential to the provision of care to the patient. In addition, their needs are as important as those of the patient.

2. Care is provided by an interdisciplinary team that assesses and provides for the patient's physical, psychological, and spiritual needs. Most patients who are followed in hospice programs are terminally ill with cancer. They do not need acute care, but rather supportive care.

3. Pain and the collateral symptoms associated with the terminal illness and its previous treatment are controlled, but no heroic efforts are made to cure the patient. In acute-care settings it is necessary for family members to request a "DNR" (do not resuscitate) order from the physician when a terminally ill person is admitted with some unrelated health problem. This is often embarrassing for the family. Yet experience has shown that codes are called on people with terminal disease who happen to enter the hospital with some other ailment unless the attending physician is requested by family members to order a "No Code." Many people are not sophisticated enough even to be aware that this option exists.

The medical board and board of directors of the Yale-New Haven Hospital have developed the following classification of approaches to the management of the terminally ill in acute-care settings:

> **Class A.** Patients are to receive all curative and functional maintenance therapies as indicated. The primary goal of care is to achieve arrest, remission, or cure of the basic disease. The aims of curative therapy take priority over those of functional maintenance, which, in turn, hold a higher priority than those of comforting therapy.
>
> **Class B.** Any curative therapy in progress is continued until its outcome is determined, and no new curative therapy is implemented. The goals of functional maintenance take priority over the goals of comforting therapy.
>
> **Class B1.** In the event of cardiopulmonary arrest the patient is to be resuscitated.
>
> **Class B2.** Do not resuscitate until order is written.
>
> **Class C.** The goals of therapy are to comfort the patient as he or she is dying. A "do not resuscitate" order is written, and comforting therapy dominates.

Curative therapies are those that are aimed at arresting or reversing the basic disease process. The aim of curative therapy is to cure the disease or to gain a remission. An underlying judgment is made by the physician that the disease is reversible. Often the iatrogenic effects of the treatments are neither considered nor disclosed to the patient and the family, or the disclosure is made in language that is difficult for them to understand. Far too often, the alternatives to one particular type of care are not disclosed, nor is the ultimate prognosis.[15]

The last basic principle on which hospice care is based is the following:

4. Bereavement follow-up is provided to the family members to help overcome their emotional suffering. This care phase is in stark contrast with the hospital setting where the survivors are most often given the clothing in a brown bag and sent home with little if any follow-up from the staff. Hospital nurses are encouraged not to attend patients' funerals and to terminate their nursing affiliation with the family once the death has occurred. Hospice provides care not only for the dying person and the family during the illness but also to the survivors after the patient's death. Thus hospice care begins with the patient's admission to the hospice program, continues to the death, and lasts for an indefinite amount of time afterwards, perhaps as long as one year. This follow-up helps the family members through the acute phases of grief and supports them during resolution. Many hospice workers who do bereavement care are people who have recently been bereaved. Thus they understand and are sensitive to the needs and feelings of those who are recently bereaved.

SUMMARY

The hospice movement arose out of a need to remove the care of the terminally ill from the acute-care setting and with the realization that death occurs in spite of technology and that the environment where death occurs need not be lonely and empty. The question "What makes hospice unique?" is answered by understanding that a hospice:

> Does not seek to cure; rather it seeks to palliate and heal.
>
> Provides care for the patient as well as care and support for the family.
>
> Provides care not only in an institutional setting but also in the home and community.
>
> Does not terminate when the patient dies but provides bereavement care to the survivors.

Hospice provides holistic, sympathetic, empathetic, personal care to the dying and their families. It is a departure from acute care, for it creates an atmosphere of spiritual meaning at a most critical phase of family life.

NOTES

[1] Robert W. Buckingham, *The Complete Hospice Guide* (New York: Harper & Row, 1983), p. 11.

[2] Mary Risley, *The House of Healing* (Garden City, N.Y.: Doubleday, 1961), pp. 21-24.

[3] R. F. Rizzo, "Hospice: Comprehensive Terminal Care," *New York State Journal of Medicine,* October 1978, p. 1902; rpt. in Buckingham, *op. cit.,* p. 3.

⁴United States General Accounting Office, *Hospice Care: A Growing Concept in the United States* (Washington, D.C.: GAO, March 6, 1979), p. 17.

⁵Thelma Ingles, "St. Christopher's Hospice," in Michael Hamilton and Helen Reid, eds., *A Hospice Handbook: A New Way to Care for the Dying* (Grand Rapids, Mich.: Eerdmans, 1980), pp. 47-49.

⁶Buckingham, *op. cit.*, p. 13.

⁷Susan Burger, "Three Approaches to Patient Care: Hospice, Nursing Homes, and Hospitals," Hamilton and Reid, *op. cit.*, p. 132.

⁸Francis McNutt, *Healing* (Notre Dame, Ind.: Ave Maria Press, 1974), pp. 161-168

⁹Sylvia A. Larch, "Pain Control in Terminal Illness," in Hamilton and Reid, *op. cit.*, pp. 75-89.

¹⁰Kenneth P. Cohen, *Hospice: Prescription for Terminal Care* (Germantown, Md.: Aspen, 1979), pp. 89-97.

¹¹*Ibid.*, p. 95.

¹²Jack M. Zimmerman, *Hospice: Complete Care for the Terminally Ill* (Baltimore: Urban & Schwarzenberg, 1981), p. 60.

¹³*Ibid.*, p. 30.

¹⁴Buckingham, *op. cit.*, pp. 16-17.

¹⁵United States General Accounting Office, *op. cit.*, p. 7.

¹⁶Robert J. Levine, "Do Not Resuscitate Decisions and Their Implementation," in Cynthia B. Wong and Judith P. Swazey, eds. *Dilemmas of Dying* (Boston: G. K. Hall, 1981), pp. 30-33.

¹⁷Cohen, *op. cit.*, p. 76.

REFERENCES

Amenta, Madalon. "Are You Cut Out for Terminal Care?" *RN,* July 1981, pp. 47-48.

Bishop, George. *Faith Healing: God or Fraud?* Los Angeles: Sherbourne Press, 1967.

Buckingham, Robert W. *The Complete Hospice Guide.* New York: Harper & Row, 1983.

Caley, Joan M., and Joan C. Westbrook. "When a Hospice Is the Answer." *Journal of Gerontological Nursing* 9 (June 1983): 344-47.

Cohen, Kenneth P. *Hospice: Prescription for Terminal Care.* Germantown, Md.: Aspen, 1979.

Hamilton, Michael, and Helen Reid. *A Hospice Handbook: A New Way to Care for the Dying.* Grand Rapids: Eerdman, 1980.

Highfield, Martha Farrar, and Carolyn Cason. "Spiritual Needs of Patients: Are They Recognized?" *Cancer Nursing,* June 1983, pp. 187-92.

Holleb, Arthur, I., ed. "Hospice Care." *Ca—A Cancer Journal for Clinicians,* 34 (July-August 1984): 178-205.

Krant, Melvin J. *Dying and Dignity: The Meaning and Control of a Personal Death.* Springfield, Ill.: Charles C. Thomas, 1974.

Krippner, Stanley, and Alberto Vivaldo. *The Realms of Healing.* Millbrae, Calif.: Celestial Arts, 1976.

Kubler-Ross, Elisabeth. *On Death and Dying.* New York: Macmillan, 1969.

Kubler-Ross, Elisabeth. *Questions and Answers on Death and Dying.* New York: Macmillan, 1974.

Kubler-Ross, Elisabeth. *Death: The Final Stage of Growth.* Englewood Cliffs, N.J.: Prentice-Hall, 1975.

Kubler-Ross, Elisabeth. *To Live Until We Say Goodbye.* Englewood Cliffs, N.J.: Prentice-Hall, 1978.

Lewis, Frances Marcus. "Family Level Services for the Cancer Patient: Critical Distinctions, Fallacies, and Assessment." *Cancer Nursing,* June 1983, pp. 193-99.

MacNutt, Francis. *Healing.* Notre Dame, Ind.: Ave Maria Press, 1974.

Naegele, Kasper D. *Health and Healing.* San Francisco: Jossey/Bass, 1970.

Prichard, Elizabeth R., Jean Collard, Janet Starr, Josephine A. Lockwood, Austin H. Kutscher, and Irene B. Seeland, eds. *Home Care: Living with Dying.* New York: Columbia University Press, 1979.

Risley, Mary. *The House of Healing.* Garden City, N.Y.: Doubleday, 1961.

Rodek, Christine F., and Susan Jacob. "Perspectives on Hospice." *Cancer Nursing,* June 1983, pp. 181-95.

Russel, Louise B. *Technology in Hospitals.* Washington, D.C.: The Brookings Institute, 1979.

Schoenberg, Bernard, Arthur C. Carr, Austin H. Kutscher, David Peretz, and Ivan K. Goldberg, eds. *Anticipating Grief.* New York: Columbia University Press, 1974.

Stoddard, Sandol. *The Hospice Movement: A Better Way of Caring for the Dying.* Briarcliff Manor, N.Y.: Stein and Day, 1978.

Thomas, Virginia Major. "Hospice Nursing: Reaping the Rewards, Dealing with Stress." *Geriatric Nursing,* January/Februrary 1983, pp. 22-27.

United States Department of Health and Human Services. *Hospice Education Program for Nurses: Modules I-II.* HHS Publication No. HRS 81-27, June 1981.

United States General Accounting Office. *Hospice Care: A Growing Concept in the United States.* Washington, D.C.: GAO, March 6, 1979.

Wallace, Grace. "Spiritual Care: A Reality in Nursing Education and Practice," *The Nurses Lamp,* 23 (November 1979): 1-4.

Wong, Cynthia B., and Judith P. Swazey, eds. *Dilemmas of Dying: Policies and Procedures for Decisions Not to Treat.* Boston: G. K. Hall, 1981.

Zimmerman, Jack M. *Hospice: Complete Care for the Terminally Ill.* Baltimore: Urban and Schwarzenberg, 1981.

Chapter 2

Organization and Administration

Mary Lou Gillespie
Karen Freeman Gartland

"Thank you for all the wonderful help you gave us during the illness and death of my mother. The nurses, the home health aides, social worker and volunteers provided us with the service and support we needed during those difficult days. We couldn't have made it without you."[1]

Statements like this one from family members lift the heart of the hospice administrator. It takes skill in organization and administration to operate a comprehensive hospice program that offers nursing, home health aides, social work, counseling, volunteer, and chaplaincy services to terminally ill patients and their families. A comprehensive hospice (1) provides medically directed multidisciplinary services, (2) provides skilled care of an appropriate nature for terminally ill patients and their families, (3) helps patients and families to live as fully as possible until death, and (4) helps relieve physical, psychological, spiritual, social, and economic symptoms that may occur during the course of the disease.[2] Patient care is provided by an interdisciplinary team consisting of physicians, nurses, social workers, homemaker or home health aides, chaplains, counselors, and volunteers. The team's emphasis is on management of pain and other symptoms associated with terminal illness.

This chapter discusses the steps involved in setting up a hospice program and describes the predominant organization structures used by hospices today. We also discuss some important administrative concerns of the hospice administrator, such as contracting with other agencies and marketing hospice services. First, however, we will briefly describe two of the concerns we see as most important to the effectiveness of a hospice program: an emphasis on home care and strong community involvement.

EMPHASIS ON HOME CARE

The first hospice in the United States, founded in New Haven, Connecticut, in 1974, began as a home care program for the terminally ill. It was this hospice's example that provided the impetus for other hospices to focus on home care as the essential component of a hospice program. The majority of hospices in the United States have recognized the importance of home care and have followed the Connecticut model either by developing a home care program or by providing home care through arrangements with a home care agency. The hospice movement in this country has been a movement toward care of the terminally ill patient at home.

Hospice's roots emerged from patients', families', and caregivers' concerns for the quality of life during terminal illness as well as patients' and families' desire to receive care and die at home. However, there has been some resistance from the established health care system to the idea that home is the appropriate place to die. It has been shown that most hospice care is provided at home. The National Hospice Project[3] funded by the federal government to study hospice care in 26 hospices across the country reported the following data on inpatient use:

> 38.9 percent of patients in hospices without inpatient beds are hospitalized an average of 5 to 6 days (represents 12.2% of duration of hospice care).
>
> 78.0 percent of patients in hospices with inpatient beds are hospitalized for an average of 17.7 days (represents 43.2% of duration of hospice care).

Data provided by the study were used to promote recent passage of the National Hospice Law.

Hospice care became reimbursible through Medicare in 1983. Home care is considered such an important component of hospice care that the Medicare regulation limits the number of inpatient days to 20 percent of the total hospice benefit days. A new hospice should focus on home care as the first priority.

There are various ways of organizing hospice care. A survey by the American Hospital Association in 1982[4] revealed the following breakdown:

> 41 percent of hospices are independent agencies licensed as home care agencies.
>
> 38 percent of hospices are hospital-based agencies that provide or arrange for home care.
>
> 18 percent of hospices are home-health-agency-based (the fastest growing group).

COMMUNITY INVOLVEMENT

Hospices emerge from the activities of special-interest groups. Many of the people who become active in initiating a hospice program had unfortunate experiences with the way a family member, friend, or patient died. The Connecticut Hospice, the Hospice of Marin in Marin County, California, the Hospice of Northern Virginia, and Hospice, Inc., in Miami, Florida, all began with special-interest groups. Such groups evolve from informal to more formal organizational structures. An example of this is the Southeast Texas Hospice in Orange, Texas. In 1974, a home care administrator, a nurse, a priest, and a community volunteer met to discuss a more humane way to care for dying people. Their initial plan of action was to attend a Kubler-Ross seminar on death and dying. This resulted in a personal visit with Dr. Elisabeth Kubler-Ross, who told them that they already had the most important ingredient for developing a hospice—an interested group. They also visited the Connecticut Hospice. Inspired, the group members tried to convince local administrators in hospitals and home health agencies to take on the hospice project, but they were not successful. However, they did find others who were willing to become involved.

The group was incorporated in 1976. They established a broad-based community board composed of a district judge, the president of a labor union, several physicians, an oil company executive, a political leader, and other influential members in the community. The board's first major activity was to raise money, each member taking an active part in speaking at hospitals, churches, social and civic club meetings, and anywhere else that people would listen. Their message was to explain the hospice project and request donations. According to Mary McKenna, administrator of the Southeast Texas Hospice, the request was, "We need your time, your prayers, and your money." Eighteen months later, $38,000 was available for their first budget year.

Then came the struggle to obtain a certificate of need for a home health agency (Texas no longer requires a certificate of need for home health). Opposing the certificate of need were three nursing homes and three large home health agency chains that maintained that they were already providing care to the terminally ill and that hospice was no different than home care. This was a common attitude in the early years and one that was supported by the state association for home health agencies at the time. Following a two-year battle, Southeast Texas Hospice received a certificate of need. The board hired an administrator, and under her leadership the agency became a Medicare-certified home health agency with the mission "care of the terminally ill and their families." The date was February 1979, and the first independent hospice in Texas began providing service, the culmination of five years of courage and persistence. Southeast Texas Hospice now serves 95 patients and families each year. The organizational structure in this case followed a pattern of developing a strong community support base, incorporating, establishing a community board, obtaining funding for the first year, applying for a certificate of need, and hiring an administrator.

HOSPICE DEVELOPMENT

Gaining Community Support

The first step for a group meeting for the purpose of developing a hospice is to gain community support by involving individuals with a personal or professional commitment to the hospice concept. Established agencies, as well as newly forming ones, need community support. One agency, the Visiting Nurse Association of Dallas, formed a special committee of administrative and supervisory staff to plan their hospice project. They involved a number of their board members, who gave the community support needed to start the project.

The second step is to provide the interest group with a more formal structure, generally a task force or planning committee. This committee can further expand the number of individuals involved by spreading information about the hospice concept through direct contact with individuals and groups. Conducting mail surveys may provide a means of stimulating interest among physicians, nurses, and other select groups. Established agencies can enlist the support of their volunteers and encourage the involvement of the members of their board and standing committees.

A third and vital step is involving the medical community. Physician support is essential for a successful hospice. Zimmerman states, "It is important to recognize that physician involvement must occur early in the planning stages. Nothing discourages physician participation faster than to be presented with a virtually fully developed protocol for a program that has been developed without physician input."[5] With the successful establishment of a community support group, a formal planning group, and involvement of the medical community, the time is right to proceed with a hospice plan and community assessment.

Assessing Community Needs and Resources

Special interest groups provide the enthusiasm and motivation that are necessary for the development of a local hospice. But it is the responsibility of the planning group to evaluate the community's need for a hospice. This group must define the service area as well as project the number of patients.

Patient access and staff travel time are primary considerations in defining the service area. It has been suggested by several health care providers that staff travel time for the home care component not exceed 30 minutes. In addition, between 60 and 90 minutes is an acceptable time for patient travel to the inpatient facility.

Since hospice is a relatively new concept of health care delivery in the United States, there is no generally accepted method of projecting the number of potential hospice patients in a community. An important index used to determine the number of hospice patients is the cancer mortality rates. One should examine both the percentage of cancer deaths and the percentage of deaths resulting from causes other than cancer within the defined service area. A survey by the National Cancer Institute[6] reported that 387,430 persons died from cancer in 1977. Sixty percent of this population was 65 years of age or older. Based on data from the National Hospice Study, it is estimated that 90 percent of hospice patients serviced in the United States had a diagnosis of cancer. However, not every terminal cancer patient is necessarily a candidate for hospice care. The number of potential hospice patients is usually estimated as 25 percent of the projected age-adjusted cancer deaths. The method used by the Cancer Subcommittee of the Physical Health Task Force[7] is as follows:

1. Determine the age-adjusted cancer death rate for the designated area (the age-adjusted rate equals 90 percent of the cancer deaths).
2. Multiply the age-adjusted cancer death rate by 25 percent to estimate the number of potential hospice patients.

Twenty-five percent of the age-adjusted cancer deaths may be an appropriate target population for the first hospice in a community. However, studies show the percentage of hospice patients to be higher when more than one hospice services an area. The Amherst Study found that Anns Haven Hospice, Denton, Texas, served 33 percent of the age-adjusted population and the Visiting Nurse Association of Dallas served an additional 26.5 percent.

After determining the number of patients in the defined service area, one must consider the daily census of the existing programs. In evaluating the average daily census, several components may be considered: monthly fluctuation, referral sources of the existing hospice programs, census limits of the programs, scope of services offered, and marketing activities.

Finally, one should examine the average length of stay in the home care components as well as in the inpatient components of the existing hospice programs. The census of any hospice program is largely dependent on the knowledge base of the community, extent of community education on hospice during the previous year, and the number of operating hospices in the community.

In addition to the community needs assessment, exploring the existing community resources and availability is vital for program planning and hospice development. Assessing available manpower, both professional staff and volunteer, can be accomplished by consulting the Bureau of Labor, local physician organizations, nursing organizations, and volunteer organizations. Other available community resource information can be obtained from the Chamber of Commerce and community councils.

Hospice service can be enhanced by collaboration with the American Cancer Society, the American Lung Association, and the American Red Cross. The latter provides special services, such as supplies for personal needs, durable medical equipment, oxygen and suction equipment, and transportation. Other health related programs, such as Meals on Wheels, homemaker services, companion or sitter services, and volunteer transportation, may be utilized by the proposed hospice program. Using existing community resources prevents duplication of costly services and allows the new hospice to concentrate on the development of other needed services.

Hospices have developed in local communities by responding to local needs and utilizing local resources. The result has been the development of a variety of hospice organizational models during the past decade.

Organizational Models

A survey by the Joint Commission on Accreditation of Hospitals in 1982 disclosed six major organizational models for hospices.

All-Volunteer Hospices. All-volunteer hospices provide care informally in conjunction with existing home health agencies and hospitals. These programs average a paid staff of 1.5 full-time equivalent positions (FTEs); the volunteer staff members include physicians, registered nurses, social workers, and other professionals. This model uses volunteers' professional skills to provide patient care and counseling. The paid staff members coordinate patient care and volunteer activities. The advantage of an all-volunteer hospice is that it has the support of the local community and numerous dedicated volunteers. Problems do arise in maintaining an adequate volunteer force and in monitoring the quality of care when using a variety of agencies for patient care. Generally, there is an inconsistent funding base. An example of the all-volunteer hospice is the Hill Country Hospice in Fredericksburg, Texas.

Case-Management Hospices. Case-management hospices work with existing home health agencies or hospitals. These programs most often provide such hospice-specific services as spiritual and bereavement counseling, social work, and volunteer services. The hospice in this instance is supplemental and is not primarily responsible for the medical care of the patient.

This model is also referred to as the "coalition" model. Hospices of this type generally have some paid staff members who receive patient referrals and coordinate patient care activities in conjunction with other agencies. They provide hospice-specific care through staff members and trained volunteers. The advantages of this model are that a number of health care agencies support the hospice, which results in good use of community resources and a broad base of community support. The disadvantages are difficulty in coordinating patient care among several agencies, difficulty in maintaining adequate numbers of volunteers, lack of consistent funding, and no third-party reimbursement. An example of the case-management model is the Lower Cape Fear Hospice, Wilmington, North Carolina.

Nursing-Home-Based Hospices. A long-term-care facility (nursing home), most often a skilled nursing facility, can provide hospice care by setting aside beds for hospice patients. Such a program may or may not have identified hospice inpatient staff members but usually provides home care services through a contract with a home care agency.

The nursing-home-model hospices are few in number. Two long-term-care-facilities received hospice grants from the National Cancer Institute to study hospice care. The facilities, Hill Haven Nursing Facility in Tucson, Arizona, and Riverside Hospice in Boontown, New Jersey, had inpatient units and home care programs. Hill Haven discontinued its hospice program in 1981. The advantage of this model is the ease with which an inpatient unit can be developed and the availability of nursing facilities in many small communities. The disadvantage is the stigma often attached to nursing homes. Current examples of this model are the Riverside Hospice, Boontown, New Jersey, and the Stella Maris Hospice in Towson, Maryland. The latter is profiled in a Case Example later in this book.

Independent Hospice Programs. Independent hospice programs, which are not owned by any other institution or agency, are usually licensed and receive reimbursement as home health agencies but serve hospice patients only. Their arrangements for hospice inpatient care are the same as outlined for home health agencies (see below). Independent hospices have their own administration and paid and volunteer staff members who provide services directly to patients and families. Inpatient care is provided in the hospice's own unit or through arrangements with a hospital. In the latter case there is close coordination between hospital and hospice to assure continuity of care for the patient and family.

The advantages of this model are several. First, the agency's mission is hospice care only. There is usually broad community support, because the hospice is not tied to a large institution, a high degree of control over all aspects of patient and family care, and high visibility in the community, which helps generate contributions. The disadvantages of this model are lack of the security that a large agency's support provides; in addition, the independent hospice must assume responsibility for all of its fund raising. Examples of independent hospices are San Diego Hospice Corporation, San Diego, California, which contracts for inpatient care; and the Hospice of Northern Virginia, Arlington, Virginia, which operates its own inpatient unit.

Hospital-Based Hospice. An acute-care hospital may maintain a hospice program that offers inpatient hospice care on one unit or on a scattered-bed approach with a floating hospice team and provides home care either by a hospital-based home health agency or through arrangements with community-based home health agencies. The acute-care hospital hospice offers inpatient care provided by trained hospice staff and volunteers. There is close coordination with the home care program. The advantages of the hospital model are continuity of care for the patient between the acute-care unit, the hospice unit, and the home care unit, well-developed quality control measures, and the financial backing of the hospital. The disadvantages are that a small program can be "lost" in a large institution, there may be low community visibility, and the hospital may impose restrictions that make implementation of hospice procedures difficult. Examples of acute care hospital settings are Community Hospice of St. Joseph's, Fort Worth, Texas, and Mercy Hospital Hospice, Rockville Centre, New York, which is described in a Case Example.

Community- or Home-Health-Agency-Based Hospices. A community health agency, most often a visiting nurse association, provides hospice home care in one of two ways: either an identified team provides hospice care only, or all staff members provide hospice care only to identified hospice patients. The program usually has informal, verbal arrangements for maintaining contact with patients when they are admitted to a hospital.

The home-health-agency-based hospice provides home care with paid professional staff and supplemental service with volunteers. All staff members and volunteers are hospice trained. The emphasis in this model is on providing care at home and on providing necessary support services to the family. The advantages to this model are well-trained, experienced home care staff, excellent community support (especially if the hospice is part of a United Way agency), a stable financial base, and generally good working relationships with hospitals and other health care organizations. The disadvantages can be competition with the agency's home care program, difficulty in implementing support systems for the hospice staff, problems related to differences in the hospice's medical and nursing care policies, and resentment of agency staff members toward the hospice staff, who they may see as receiving special care and recognition. Examples of this model are the Visiting Nurse Association of Dallas Home Hospice Program, Dallas, Texas, and the hospice program of the Home Nursing Agency, Altoona, Pennsylvania, which is profiled latter in this book.

Home-health-agency-based hospices and independent hospices are increasing in number. The home-health-agency-based and freestanding hospices certified by Medicare have formal contracts with hospitals for inpatient care or open their own inpatient units, such as was done by Hospice, Inc., Miami, Florida, a home hospice program with a hospice inpatient unit in a local acute care hospital maintained through a leased-space agreement.

ORGANIZATIONAL STRUCTURES

Most formal hospice planning groups make early decisions regarding organizational structures for their hospice programs. Incorporation is the first step toward a formal organizational structure. Decisions on incorporation, tax status, and agency mission are usually made prior to filing the incorporation application.

In some states there are laws mandating that home health agencies be nonprofit. The nonprofit agency has the advantages of receiving tax deductible donations, grants, and foundation monies, possibly qualifying for United Way affiliation, and being viewed as a charitable organization. The major disadvantages for the nonprofit agency are lack of money for program expansion, little incentive to raise funds for needed services, low staff salaries, and often a non-business-oriented board. Nonprofit agencies can use excess revenues for program expansion, but the reality for most nonprofit hospices is that there are rarely any excess revenues.

If state law permits it, for-profit tax status is an option open to planning groups. For-profit hospices are few in number, and most of them are part of for-profit hospitals. There seems to be a belief among many hospice administrators that hospices should be nonprofit. Often there is an assumption that for-profit agencies take only paying patients and that their emphasis is on making money; therefore they feel that nonprofit status contradicts the basic philosophy of hospice care.

The advantages of the for-profit status are that adequate start-up funds can be secured through private investors, the hospice can attract experienced business people, and a charity fund can be established, making the limited charity dollars in the community go further. The first company to develop a for-profit charity fund is Hospice Care, Inc., of Miami, Florida, whose first for-profit hospice unit is located in Dallas, Texas (Dallas Hospice Care, Inc.).

Once the decision on tax status has been made, the planning group must develop bylaws, which include the agency's purpose or mission statement. The mission of a hospice program can be stated in one sentence, such as, "To provide care to terminally ill persons and their families," or it can be expanded to include the type of care, by whom it is delivered, and in what location. Either description of the hospice concept or the National Hospice Organization definition of a hospice program are appropriate mission statements. Established agencies that set up hospice programs must give thought to writing separate mission statements for their hospices.

Other factors to consider in planning the hospice organizational structure are Medicare reimbursement, licensure and certificate of need laws, and the size of the hospice. Generally, independent, hospital-based, and home-health-agency-based hospices desire Medicare certification.

Medicare Reimbursement

In 1983, Medicare began providing benefits to eligible patients of hospices that could meet strict eligibility requirements. Among the most important requirements are: 1) the hospice must be an identifiable unit with one individual responsible for its day-to-day management, 2) the hospice staff must be designated, and personnel records and budgets must reflect this, 3) hospice must provide nursing care directly, 4) volunteers must provide services to the hospice equaling at least 5 percent of direct patient care hours. The simplest way for an established agency to meet Medicare requirements is to set up the hospice as a subunit of a home health agency.

However, there are hospices that do not seek Medicare reimbursement in order to avoid the restrictions of the Medicare regulations, even though they are licensed as home health agencies. Medicare reimbursement does enable hospices to provide more services to both Medicare beneficiaries and other patients, as Medicare reimbursement allows more of the agency's charitable contributions to be made available to non-Medicare patients. (See Chapter 3 for a more detailed explanation of the Medicare regulations and their advantages and disadvantages for hospice programs.)

Licensure. In order to receive Medicare reimbursement, a hospice must be licensed by the state as a hospice or home health agency. The decision to become a licensed home health agency usually coincides with the decision to seek Medicare certification. As of May 1984, fifteen states have hospice licensure laws. In addition to licensure laws, some states require a certificate of need for home health or hospice licensure. Obtaining a certificate of need may take considerable time and money. Merging with an agency that already has a certificate of need can be a cost-effective strategy.

The decision to open an inpatient unit in conjunction with a hospice home care program adds another dimension to the organizational structure. A free-standing hospice inpatient unit might be licensed as a special hospital, an acute-care hospital, or a skilled nursing facility. However, it may not be necessary for hospital-based hospices to obtain separate licenses for inpatient units within the hospital, unless state laws require it.

Size of Agency

The size of the agency and the projected number of hospice patients affect the organizational structure. In a large VNA with a potential patient population of 600 to 800 patients a year, the hospice might be either a separate program with its own administrator or a subunit of the home care program with the home care administrator giving an appropriate number of hours to the hospice service. In a moderate-sized hospice serving 100 to 300 patients per year, an appropriate structure would be a subunit of the home care program with designated part-time management staff. The small-sized hospice, often in a rural area or small town, that serves 50 to 100 patients per year, might be a small unit within a home health agency or hospital that uses part-time staff or shares staff members and uses many volunteers.

There are a number of small, independent hospices with an administrator who directs the total operation and sometimes supervises caregivers, especially if the administrator is a registered nurse. The administrator is often the only management person on staff.

FINANCING THE HOSPICE

Starting a hospice program takes money, whether it is planned as a new independent hospice or as a program within an established agency or hospital. Functioning within a licensed and accredited institution may provide freedom and protection to the hospice.[8] In addition, the parent agency often has available space, utilities, and administrative and clerical staff. Both hospitals and home health agencies, especially if they are nonprofit, may have access to funds from local foundations and grants. For example, the Visiting Nurse Association of Dallas received start-up money for its hospice program through grants from the King Foundation and the Junior League. In addition, United Way agreed to the use of United Way dollars for hospice.

Raising money for start up is difficult. Start up begins at the point an administrator is hired. Fund raising causes a dilemma for planning groups, because money is needed before service is available—and the consumer needs care *now*. The planning group is caught in a dilemma—by providing information to the public, they increase the demand for service, yet the hospice cannot offer services. The group can respond to the demand for service by using volunteers to provide care or by referring patients to a home health agency. The kind of service provided or coordinated by the hospice group must be good, as a few bad publicity reports can affect a group's ability to raise money in the community.

The start-up dollars pay for staff salaries and benefits, rental of space, utilities, office supplies and equipment, travel, and insurance. The time from the start-up point to service delivery averages 6 to 12 months for most new hospices. It is expected that the hospice will operate in the red for the first year, if it relies primarily on third-party reimbursement. The point at which revenues meet expenses varies as much as do the organizational structures of hospices. A reasonable expectation for a moderate or large hospice is one year.

Projecting revenues for a Medicare-certified hospice, keeping in mind prospective reimbursement, involves the following factors: percentage of hospice patients that are Medicare eligible, percentage of Medicaid-eligible patients, the state Medicaid coverage for hospice, percentage of private-insurance patients, percentage of private-pay and part-pay patients, and estimated amount of donations, grants, and United Way funding.

ADMINISTRATIVE STRUCTURES

The administrative structure and line of authority within an organization are determined by agency ownership. Visiting nurse associations are nonprofit community agencies with volunteer policy-making boards of directors. The board members donate their time and have the responsibility for setting agency policy, monitoring finances and service delivery and hiring the executive director. The board of directors often delegates program review and evaluation to advisory committees. These committees may make recommendations to the board of directors for policy changes within programs they oversee, but the board of directors reviews and votes on all changes.

The home health agency or home hospice that is privately owned and nonprofit is administered by an executive board, usually consisting of the owners, a treasurer, and a secretary. The agency sets up volunteer advisory committees for special activities, such as utilization review, personnel, volunteers, and so forth. The hospice that is for-profit and privately owned operates much the same way as the nonprofit. However, there is a difference in for-profit hospices funded by private investors; the corporate board members dictate policy even though much of the work is done by the executive committee of the corporate board, and advisory committees are used for special activities (review of medical policies, marketing, and community education).

The lines of authority are best illustrated by the organizational charts of a hospice in a VNA, a privately owned nonprofit hospice, and a privately owned for-profit hospice.

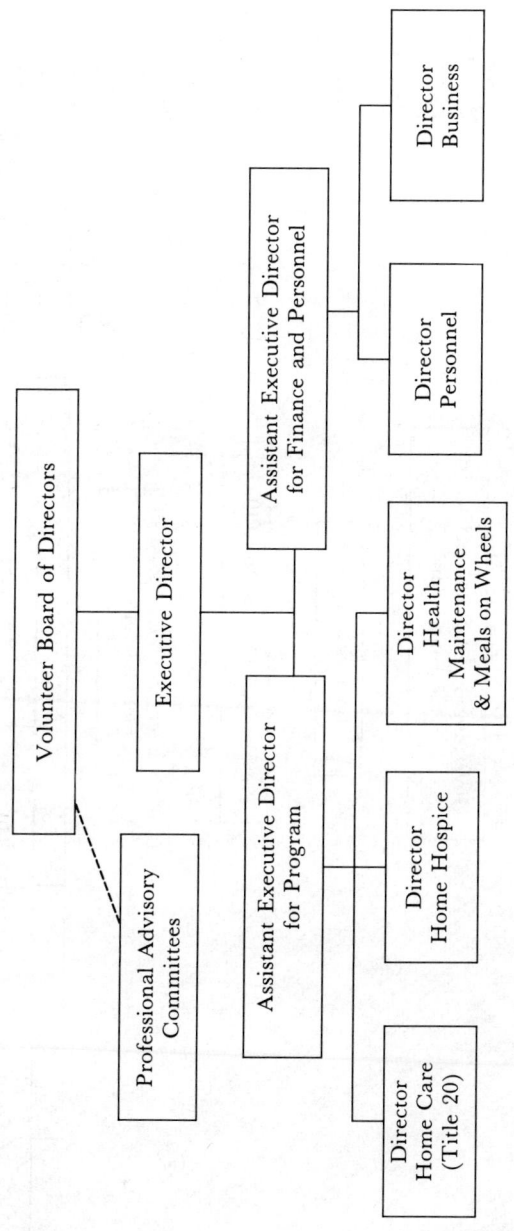

Figure 2.1 Visiting Nurse Association of Dallas, 1979-80

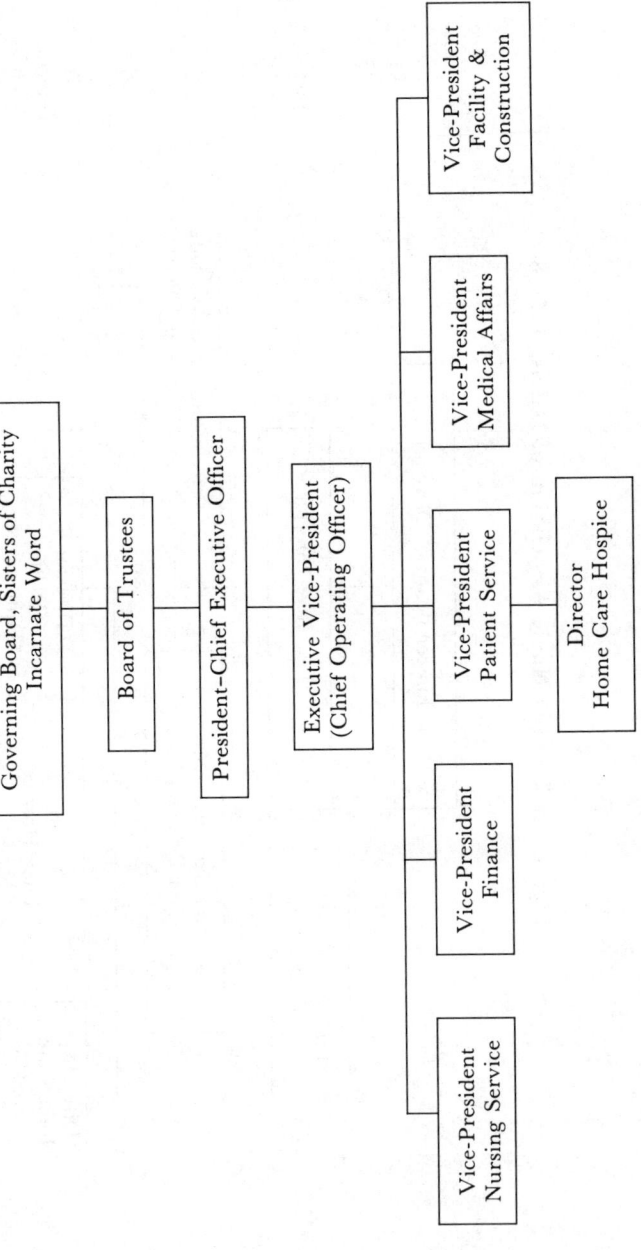

Figure 2.2 Community Hospice of St. Joseph, Ft. Worth

Figure 2.3 Dallas Hospice Care, Inc.

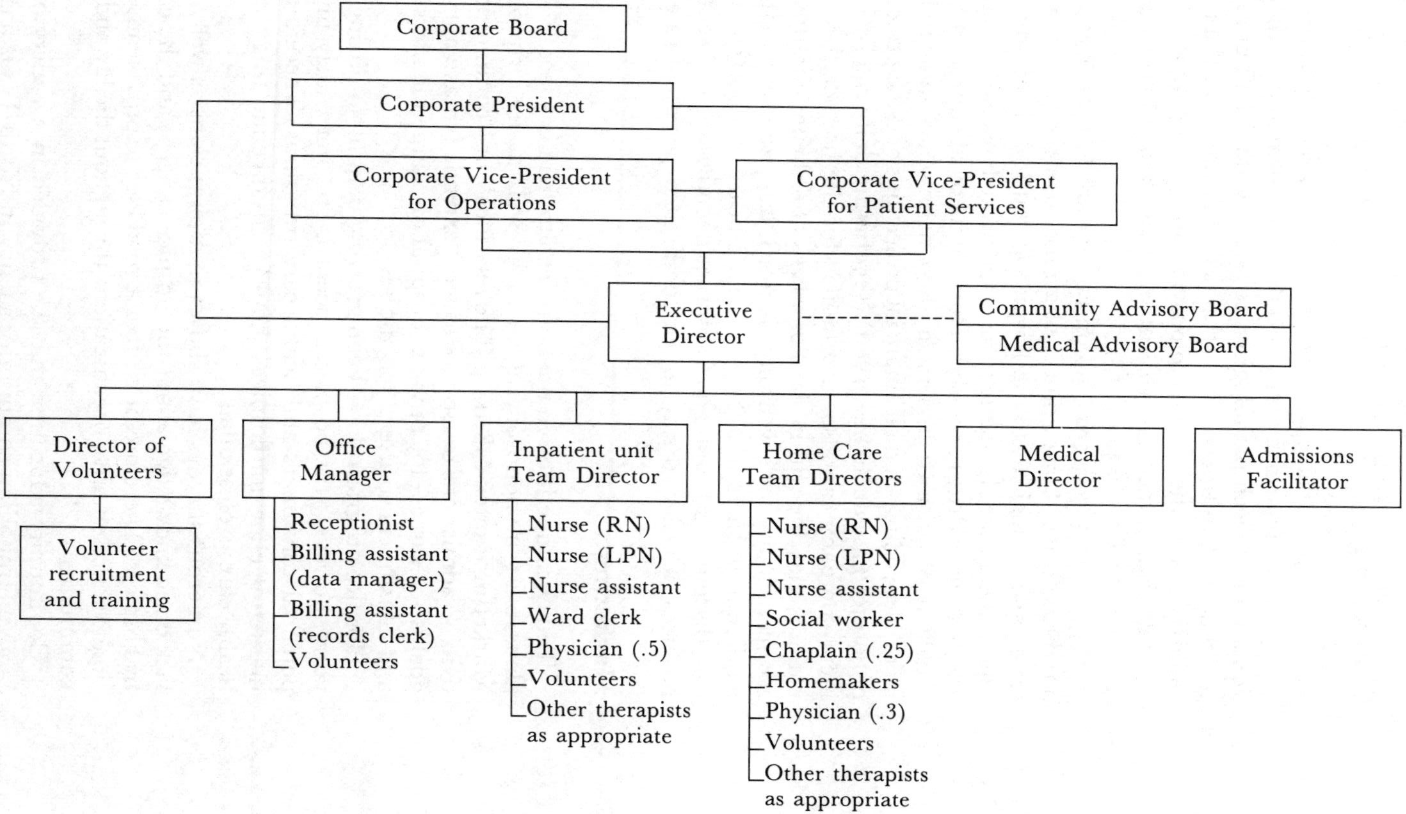

- Corporate Board
  - Corporate President
    - Corporate Vice-President for Operations
    - Corporate Vice-President for Patient Services
      - Executive Director ---- Community Advisory Board / Medical Advisory Board
        - Director of Volunteers
          - Volunteer recruitment and training
        - Office Manager
          - Receptionist
          - Billing assistant (data manager)
          - Billing assistant (records clerk)
          - Volunteers
        - Inpatient unit Team Director
          - Nurse (RN)
          - Nurse (LPN)
          - Nurse assistant
          - Ward clerk
          - Physician (.5)
          - Volunteers
          - Other therapists as appropriate
        - Home Care Team Directors
          - Nurse (RN)
          - Nurse (LPN)
          - Nurse assistant
          - Social worker
          - Chaplain (.25)
          - Homemakers
          - Physician (.3)
          - Volunteers
          - Other therapists as appropriate
        - Medical Director
        - Admissions Facilitator

Contracting

A comprehensive hospice program contracts for a variety of services, such as pharmacy, physical therapy, occupational therapy, nutritionists and speech pathologists, temporary staff, and durable medical equipment. Contracts with acute-care hospitals and skilled nursing facilities enable the hospice to provide appropriate inpatient care when a patient is in a medical crisis or when the family needs a short respite from caring for the patient.

The primary concerns in contracting are to obtain good service at a reduced price. For instance, pharmacy owners may be willing to sell drugs and biologicals to the hospice at state Medicaid reimbursement rates if the hospice is willing to keep the procedures and paperwork simple and if generic drugs are used. Durable medical equipment owners will usually negotiate a 10-20 percent discount on rental and purchased equipment, depending on their financial projections and the projected number of hospice patients to be served. Negotiating daily rates with an equipment company can also save money for the hospice, because hospice patients may die within days or weeks after being admitted to hospice service. Paying for seven days is much less expensive than paying for a full month. In view of the current Medicare reimbursement rates, getting discounts through good contract negotiations is essential for most hospices in order to stay under the limited per diem rate of $46.25.

Marketing

Today competition in the home health field is a fact, and marketing plans exist in nonprofit agencies as well as in for-profit agencies. Marketing is often called "public relations" or "community liaison activity," admissions nurses are called "extended intake nurses," but the goal is the same—to convince hospital discharge planners, physicians, and consumers to use a specific service.

Hospice programs have been growing in number during the past two years; however, the hospice concept is still not widely understood by potential consumers and health care programs. Therefore, the initial marketing effort for hospices should focus on educating consumers and health care professionals.

Numerous surveys have shown that physicians as well as consumers lack basic knowledge about the hospice concept and the care provided by hospices. Therefore, it is often a good idea to provide inservice education to representative organizations throughout the lay and professional community.

Community education may be provided in a variety of ways. One large metropolitan community agency in North Texas has successfully used radio, TV, newspaper, and magazine coverage. After a newspaper article with an accompanying photograph of a hospice patient and nurse, the referrals to that agency increased significantly over a period of approximately two months. In Dallas, Texas, the local *P.M. Magazine* television show did a ten-minute special on hospice care, and the flood of telephone calls to the hospice program was beyond the agency's expectations. The hospice concept has an emotional appeal that newspaper editors and television and radio station managers are willing to promote.

Marketing the hospice's services has to be a continuing effort with emphasis on the hospice's quality and special services, such as medical-directed interdisciplinary teams, home visits by a hospice physician, homelike inpatient unit, hospice nurses making death pronouncements (if the state allows it), and 24-hour on-call nurses, physicians, and counselors.

Hospice's promise to the consumer is assurance and support during the last days or months of life. Perhaps Dame Cecily Saunders provides the best description: "You matter, because you are you. You matter to the last moment of your life, and we will do all we can—not only to help you die peacefully, but also to live until you die. To live until death, not merely exist in pain and isolation, but to live as fully as possible. Given a choice, most people with a terminal illness do not want extensive life support systems. Most people would prefer to die at home, in familiar surroundings with loved ones close by."[9]

SUMMARY

The diversity of organizational structures among hospices gives local planning groups a variety of models to consider, but because home care is included in all hospice models, home care should be the focus of the fledgling program. Clearly the success of a hospice depends on the involvement of local community members and on local funding. Tax status and administrative structure do not directly affect the quality of the hospice service. Medicare certification can make a financial difference; even though many consider the hospice Medicare regulations restrictive, Medicare provides an excellent benefit package to the beneficiaries and will bring in revenues to the hospice.

The hospice movement began with the desire of health care workers to make a difference for the dying person and grew to become a complex delivery system. The phenomenal growth of hospice in the past two years could mean that in the future hospice will be an option of care for all terminally ill patients and their families. The hospice "movement" as such may end, and hospice service will be the accepted method of care at the end of a person's life, well integrated into this country's health care system.

NOTES

[1] Excerpt from a personal letter to hospice administrator, Visiting Nurse Association of Dallas Home Hospice Program, 1981.

[2] Robert W. Buckingham, *The Complete Hospice Guide* (New York: Harper & Row, 1983), p. 73.

[3] HCFA, *National Hospice Study: Preliminary Final Report,* Grant #99-P-9779 3/1-0, (Washington, D.C.: HCFA, November 1983).

[4] Ellen A. Pyrgga and Henry J. Bachelor, *Working Paper: Hospice Care under Medicare* (Chicago: American Hospital Association, Office of Public Policy, June 1983), appendix p. 2.

[5] Jack Zimmerman, *Hospice: Complete Care for the Terminally Ill* (Baltimore: Urban and Schwarzenburg, 1981), p. 158.

[6] Cancer Subcommittee of the Physical Health Task Force, *Guidelines for the Design and Implementation of Hospice Care* (Texas Area 5 Health Systems Agency, July 15, 1980), appendix A.

[7] *Ibid.*

[8] Zimmerman, *op.cit.,* p. 41.

[9] Buckingham, *op.cit.,* p. 12.

REFERENCES

Amherst Associates, Inc., *The Visiting Nurse Association of Dallas Hospice Feasibility Study,* Dallas: Amherst Associates, June 1983.

Blum, Henrick L. *Planning for Health Development and Application of Social Change Theory.* New York: Health Science Press, 1979.

Buckingham, Robert W. *The Complete Hospice Guide* (New York: Harper & Row, 1983).

Cancer Subcommittee of the Physical Health Task Force. *Guidelines for the Design and Implementation of Hospice Care.* Texas Area 5 Health Systems Agency, July 15, 1980.

Cohen, Kenneth P. *Hospice: Prescription for Terminal Care.* Rockville, Md.: Aspen, 1979.

Corr, Charles, and Donna M. Corr. *Hospice Care: Principles and Practice.* New York: Springer, 1983.

HCFA. *National Hospice Study: Preliminary Final Report.* Grant #99-P-9779 3/1-0. Washington, DC.: HCFA, November 1983.

Zimmerman, Jack. *Hospice: Complete Care for the Terminally Ill.* Baltimore: Urban and Schwarzenburg, 1981.

Chapter 3

Reimbursement Issues

S. Jill Schultz

The financing of hospice care has been a problem from the inception of hospice services in the United States. Davidson, in his "Five Models for Hospice Care," states that the prevalence of the volunteer model is indicative of the lack of consistent funding sources.[1] Program complexity ranges from all-volunteer services with minimal cost to more complex organizations, whether temporary or permanent. Indeed there is speculation that a consistent funding source leads to a predominance of paid staff and the consequent disuse of volunteers in hospice programs.

Lack of funding was one of the factors that prevented early integration of hospice services into the traditional health care system. In the early 1970s, the scope of hospice services was limited by the availability of health professional volunteers.[2] In the United States the Connecticut Hospice in New Haven and the Hospice of Marin in California relied on services of established home health agencies for skilled care and provided symptom control and psychosocial support through the hospice program.[3] Freestanding facilities were not developed until nontraditional funding sources were found.[4]

Before the enactment of the Medicare hospice benefit in the Tax Equity and Fiscal Responsibility Act (TEFRA) of 1982, hospice programs had few sources of funds, because hospice was not considered a single entity reimbursable under any third-party insurer. Hospice programs had to depend on philanthropy and temporary funds from other sources. Services were funded through donations, memorials, membership fees, private and public grants, and other fund-raising activities. In spite of Medicare reimbursement, however, many programs must still rely on these sources to pay for services that are not reimbursable through entitlement funds. In addition, because of problems inherent in the Medicare regulations, many hospices have chosen not to seek Medicare certification.

Fund raising in the community was aided by the emotional appeal of the hospice concept. Publicity about hospice programs appeals to both consumers and health care professionals.

Families and friends of the dying are often the best fund raisers for a hospice program, bringing in small but important donations and memorial contributions. Few hospice programs can afford professional fund raisers; therefore volunteers with little or no fund-raising experience are used. Depending on their expertise, fund raising varies from occasional donations to sophisticated fund raising techniques.

Hospices often solicit members, both individual and institutional, in order to involve interested members of the public in their activities. The individual membership fee is usually nominal and may include voting privileges or newsletter subscriptions. Institutional membership is more expensive and often entitles the institution to board membership.

Administrators of health agencies noted the popularity of hospice programs and quickly sought to become members of the board, if only to keep informed of the program's development, which can influence their own institutions. The positive public relations created by the hospice programs provides an incentive for traditional health care providers to become associated with the movement, in this way. In addition, board members from the financial community are valued for their contacts and their knowledge.

Community United Way funds are sought by hospice providers either as a separate program or as a program of an existing United Way agency. In addition to availability of funds, the underwriting of hospice services by United Way also depends on admission criteria for United Way affiliates and on the local United Way's position on hospice programs. In addition, hospice providers must consider the impact that established United Way fund raising and financial accountability policies can have on the total program.

Foundation funds have been a source of hospice operating funds and capital funds. While these funds vary in size, purpose, and duration, most foundations prefer short-term funding over long-term and therefore are not considered stable sources of funds. Hillhaven Foundation is an example of a foundation that is funding a hospice program;[5] the National Cancer Institute funded several hospice programs in the mid-1970s, including the Connecticut Hospice.[6]

In addition to fund raising and foundation funds, partial costs of hospice programs are often met by Federal entitlement programs, such as Titles 18 and 20. Funds are secured from other sources for noncovered costs.

To meet their costs, hospice programs develop liaisons with a variety of existing providers or merge with a larger agency. A hospital involved in the development of a hospice program may extend hospice services under its own auspices. Because home care is a vital part of a hospice program, the hospital either develops linkages with an existing home care provider[7] or seeks certification as a home health agency. Community-based hospices, which were developed by a variety of health-institution representatives and lay community participants, were pressured as their programs evolved to seek a means of financial stability. The most common route was to become a home care provider. This ensured that at least some of the program's costs could be recovered. (See the Case Examples on community- and hospital-based hospice programs.) Affiliation with nursing home providers is another means of meeting some costs and, in addition, of potentially increasing the nursing home's occupancy.[8] Wholly volunteer programs that can no longer meet the demand for services are faced with the decision either to limit services or to consider affiliation with an existing health care provider.

Blue Cross/Blue Shield programs in several states have provided funds for the operation of hospice programs to establish a data base on hospice care. For example, Blue Cross/Blue Shield of Michigan funded several programs in order to (1) identify and estimate the demand for hospice care in the Blue Cross target population (under age 65), (2) compare the costs of care for those in a hospice program with costs for those outside the program, and (3) determine the quality of life or how hospice recipients perceive the hospice benefit. The latter objective was dispensed with because of a lack of adequate evaluation tools.[9]

The purpose of collecting cost data was to determine the potential extent of Blue Cross/Blue Shield financial liability and other third-party liability, the size of out-of-pocket costs, and the total cost per episode of terminal illness. The models included in the study were hospice inpatient care, hospice home care, and the traditional method of care. Reimbursement for the services varied from payment of individual cases to payment based on the proportion of the target population the Blue Cross/Blue Shield plan served. After the two-year period of data collection, the researchers concluded that costs were generally highest in the inpatient hospice model. The greatest concern of all potential reimbursers of hospice services was that the cost of hospice care would not replace traditional costs for terminal illness, but would in effect be an add-on to already high health care costs. The results of the study were equivocal in that existence of a "substitution effect" was not substantiated, but neither was cost reduction.

The U.S. Department of Health and Human Services, through the Health Care Financing Administration (HCFA), established a demonstration project that funded a cross-section of hospice programs. The demonstration project collected data only on persons 65 years of age and older and paid all costs of the programs for the sample patients.

Neither the Blue Cross/Blue Shield pilot programs nor the HCFA demonstration projects conclusively demonstrated that hospice services were used either as a substitute for traditional care or as an add-on. In spite of the uncertainty of the costs involved, the Medicare hospice benefit had already been legislated, and HCFA began to propose and implement regulations.

THE MEDICARE REGULATIONS—TEFRA 1982

The passage of the Medicare hospice benefit has been claimed to be the result of the political astuteness of the hospice movement leadership. The hospice movement has been considered to resemble a crusade, and the speed of the enactment of the legislation has been said to demonstrate the fervor created in legislators by hospice supporters.

Hospice providers view the passage of the legislation as a victory for the hospice concept. However, since the implementation of the rules and regulations, many have felt that the victory may be short-lived.[10] Of the estimated 1,200 hospice programs in the United States, less than 10 percent have sought certification,[11] and hospice providers have voiced their opposition to the required direct provision of core services and to the reimbursement rates and procedures.[12] Direct opposition to these provisions continues in Congress.

There is some speculation that the rules and regulations were developed to undermine the usefulness of the hospice benefit,[13] as it was perceived by HFCA as a cost added to the already burdened health care system. The legislation itself is said to be exactly what the hospice leadership intended; however, its interpretation by HCFA appears to be the problem.[14] The following sections provide a brief overview of the hospice regulations and the problems and issues they raise.

Rules and Regulations

The final rules and regulations for the Medicare hospice benefit were published in the *Federal Register* of December 16, 1983. HCFA maintains that these were written using the findings of the 26 demonstration projects. The rules spelled out the responsibilities and requirements of both the patient and the provider.

The Patient. The patient's participation in the program depends on meeting the eligibility criteria, which consist of the following:

1. Medicare eligibility.
2. Terminally ill status with less than 6 months to live.

3. Prognosis certified by the attending physician (the physician who has the most significant role in the patient's care at the time he elects hospice care).

The patient must elect hospice care. In doing so, he waives his right to traditional (curative) Medicare benefits.

The patient is entitled to two 90-day periods of hospice services, plus one 30-day period in his lifetime. The services include physician services, nursing, therapy services, counseling, specialty physician services, home health aide services, homemaker services, medical supplies, short-term inpatient care, and bereavement counseling for the family.

The Provider. Hospice providers certified under Medicare must meet the following conditions:

1. Provide core home-care services (nursing, medical-social services, physician services, and counseling) directly, not through subcontracts.
2. Maintain professional management of the patient when services are provided through contracts with inpatient institutions.
3. Establish and maintain a written plan of care.
4. Continue care even after the patient exhausts the hospice benefit.
5. Inform the hospice patient of his rights under the hospice program.
6. Provide an ongoing inservice education program for employees.
7. Evaluate care given on an ongoing basis.
8. Provide care through the workings of an interdisciplinary group of health care providers.
9. Employ volunteers and maintain records on volunteer services.
10. Comply with state and local laws.
11. Maintain central clinical records.
12. Provide other (noncore) services either directly or by means of contracts with other agencies.
13. Contract for inpatient short-term care as needed (with the provision that no more than 20 percent of care be provided on an inpatient basis; this is the so-called 80/20 rule).
14. Obtain state approval of the hospice program and provider agreements.

State agencies are to determine a hospice's compliance with the conditions of participation.

Reimbursement

Coverage falls under Medicare Part A, except when the attending physician is not a hospice medical director, in which case coverage is under Medicare Part B. Payment for services is on a prospective basis, according to the published rules and regulations: hospices are paid a predetermined rate for each day a Medicare beneficiary is under the care of the hospice program. However, there is a cap on reimbursement for each patient of $6,500 for any twelve-month period, and, as shown in the next section, there are aspects of the regulations that make the system a combination of prospective and retrospective reimbursement.

The predetermined rates are:

1. Routine home care: $46.25 per day.
2. Continuous home care: $358.67 per day.
3. Eight hours of home care: $119.56 per day; $14.94 per hour, each additional hour thereafter.
4. Inpatient respite care: $55.33 per day.
5. General inpatient care: $271.00 per day.

Average rates are given here. All home care rates will be adjusted on the basis of the local wage index. According to HCFA, reimbursement rates were established based on data collected during the hospice demonstration projects.

Issues

Features of the hospice benefit that trouble most potential providers include, but are not limited to, the following:

1. Direct core services provision.
2. The reimbursement rates themselves and the way they are administered.
3. Hospice accountability for all professional and financial management of services.

Direct Core Services Provision. Core services to be provided directly by the hospice program include nursing services, medical social services, physicians' services, and counseling. The inability to subcontract for core services alarmed rural hospices in particular, since they often subcontract for nursing services because of their small caseloads and lack of available personnel. To provide the services directly or restructure the hospice program will increase their costs.

HCFA chief Carolyne Davis defended the direct care provision because not to provide direct care, she stated, would be "inconsistent with the hospice concept."[15] However, testimony submitted by the National Association of Home Care (NAHC) stated that without a change in the provision many rural hospices would not participate in the hospice benefit.[16]

Home health agencies viewed the direct-care provision as a means of eliminating their participation in hospice programs and reducing their caseload of terminal patients, arguing that they had provided care to the terminally ill before the hospice movement began and were being forced to discontinue to do so. The rule that hospices must provide direct core services was a sign to home health agencies that the National Hospice Organization (NHO) leadership did not want to share any territory with home health agencies. NHO denied that it intended to exclude home health agencies and published the NHO hospice monograph, a how-to pamphlet describing how to structure a hospice and home health agency relationship to meet the core service requirement for nursing care.[17]

The inclusion of the core services provision has created controversy. The search for resolution through legislation continues at the time of this writing.

Reimbursement Rates. The rates established in the *Federal Register* are based on data collected in the HCFA demonstration projects. However, many of the hospices feel they cannot remain financially viable at these rates. The rates assumed an average length of stay of 70 days. Conditions of participation require that no more than 20 percent of the total number of days of Medicare hospice care be provided on an inpatient basis and that reimbursement not exceed $6,500 per patient within a twelve-month period.

However, several different combinations of types of care, with different rates of reimbursement, are possible, as the following examples illustrate. All of the examples are based on the average 70 days of care and the maximum allowable 20 percent of days of inpatient care.

Patient A

56 days of routine home care ($46.25)	=	$ 2,590
14 days of inpatient respite care ($55.33)	=	774
Total cost		$ 3,364

Patient B

56 days at eight hours of care per day ($119.56)	=	$ 6,695
14 days of inpatient care ($271.00)	=	3,794
Total cost		$10,489

Patient C

56 days of continuous home care ($358.67)	=	$20,085
14 days of inpatient care ($271.00)	=	3,794
Total cost		$23,879

The reimbursement rate varies for these three patients from a low of $3,364 to a high of $23,879 per case. The cap amount of $6,500 could easily be exceeded; on the other hand, cases in which minimal services were required could certainly make a profit.

The potential for inadequate reimbursement for complex cases is relatively simple to grasp. There are other potential problems caused by the complexity of the methods used to determine reimbursement. Although the system purports to be a prospective payment system, it incorporates features of a retrospective payment system. One such is the so-called aggregate clause, covering hospices whose number of inpatient days for a given year is lower than 20 percent of the total days of care; cases that fall below the "80/20 rule." These hospices are retrospectively reimbursed an additional amount, which is determined as follows.

The example here, for the sake of simplicity, is based on two patients. Assume that the hypothetical agency has cared for only these two patients and therefore has a total of 100 patient days for the year, 10 for Patient D and 90 for Patient E:

Patient D—10 Days of Care

8 days of routine home care ($46.25)	=	$370.00
2 days of inpatient care ($271.00)	=	542.00
Total charges		$912.00

Patient E—90 Days of Care

79 days of routine home care ($46.25)	=	$3,653
11 days of inpatient care ($271.00)	=	2,981
Total charges		$6,634

Note that Patient E's care costs more than the Medicare cap of $6,500. Initial reimbursement for this patient would be only $6,500, whereas reimbursement for Patient D would be the full cost of $912. However, because the agency fell below the 80/20 rule for the year (total inpatient days were 13, or 13 percent of the total of 100 patient days), it is entitled to an additional, retrospective reimbursement under the aggregate clause. At the end of the year the hospice would be retrospectively reimbursed the full amount of $6,634 for Patient E, because its inpatient days were less than 20 percent of the total. On the other hand, if the hospice exceeds the 80/20 rule in the aggregate, it can owe money to Medicare at the end of the year when all cases are combined in the manner described above.

Another potential area of concern for hospices is the calculation of reimbursement for continuous home care, which is done on an area-wide basis, not on the basis of the particular hospice. The calculation is done as follows:

Step 1: Divide the number of hours of continuous home care provided by the agency by 24. This figure is the number of days of continuous home care.

Step 2: Divide the total allowable Medicare reimbursement for inpatient acute care in your area by the number of days of acute care given by hospitals in your area. This is the average daily rate of inpatient care for your area.

Step 3: Multiply the result of Step 2 by the result of Step 1. This is the number of days for which the hospice will be reimbursed for continuous home care.

Again, this is a form of retrospective payment based on complicated yearly aggregate calculations rather than per-case reimbursement. The regulations leave unclear how these figures, such as area-wide allowable reimbursement, will be determined or who will determine them. Many people believe that the purpose of the continuous home care (CHC) rule is to reduce the number of CHC hours for which hospices bill Medicare.

Other problems inherent in the Medicare regulations are the lack of a mechanism to appeal the set rates, and provision of medical supplies and respite care on a coinsurance basis, and no yearly adjustment for bad debts.

Professional and Financial Responsibility for Services. A certified hospice program, regardless of who actually provides services under its auspices, is responsible for the professional management and financing of the services. When inpatient care is provided under arrangements with other agencies, the hospice must still be the active manager of the patient's care. Reimbursement for the care is made by the hospice to the inpatient provider.

The hospice's responsibility for all care provided not only raises the possibility of legal challenge to the hospice because of malpractice by another institution but also may increase the cost of providing services. Contract negotiations are time-consuming at best, and the detail required by the regulations will increase the cost. In addition, the requirements for documentation of the hospice services adds to the cost of the program.[19]

To participate in the hospice program the patient must sign a waiver of traditional services. All services related to the terminal illness are then covered under the hospice benefit; the patient does, however, continue to receive benefits for other conditions under Medicare.

The responsibilities entailed by these provisions have raised legal and ethical questions. The patient's consent to waive traditional treatment presumes several things: (1) that the patient understands the nature of hospice, (2) that the patient understands what traditional system services are available, and (3) that the patient and family know what services they want and need.

Informed consent is an important ethical and legal issue throughout the health care field today, and the problems involved cannot be discussed at length here. For the potential hospice patient, whose cultural conditioning leads him to believe that medicine can cure anything, waiving all rights to traditional medical treatment may seem like a sentence of death. The patient may view the hospice itself as the cause of his terminal condition. In addition, physicians have great difficulty in determining the remaining length of life for terminal patients unless it is very brief, so patients may not be admitted to hospice until they have only a few days to live.

In addition, some of the regulations provide incentives that are not consistent with the hospice concept. The areas of conflict involve the way volunteers are to be used, medical direction, and incentives to limit care. Volunteers for hospice services are considered by the Medicare regulations to be employees. This raises legal and financial questions regarding the employer–employee relationship. The number of volunteers to be used in order to be certified under Medicare is unclear, and the fact that services are reimbursable could lead to a decline in the use of volunteers.

Under the regulations, medical direction is provided by the hospice medical director. The primary physician continues to provide services through traditional reimbursement. However, the hospice medical director must approve the care to be provided and the level of care. Admission for inpatient care also requires approval of the medical director. The potential for conflict between the medical director and primary physician clearly exists.

Reimbursement rates provide incentives to admit patients based on an expected short length of stay, to limit inpatient care, and to limit the amount of care to be provided.

One final problem to be mentioned here is that certification of hospice programs is the responsibility of the state in which the hospice program operates. Thus interpretation and enforcement of the regulations may vary from state to state. Such is the situation of home health care regulations.

Medicare reimbursement for hospice services has the potential to provide hospice programs with a degree of financial stability. While the benefit has a "sunset" limitation, there is the possibility that it will continue. Enactment of the legislation has been followed by an increase in the number of other third-party reimbursers that provide hospice coverage. Therefore, the increase in the number of insurance carriers covering hospice services could prevent hospice programs from becoming Medicare-only programs.

CONCLUSIONS

The funding status of hospice services in the future will depend on whether hospice care is found to reduce health care costs and whether it retains its positive public appeal. The future survival of hospice programs that do not seek Medicare certification will depend on the strength and perseverance of their volunteers and on the ability of communities to support the services.

The financing of health care services, in general, will probably change radically in the next few years. Different methods of reimbursement for services are being explored and continued efforts will be made to reduce costs. If hospice services are not viewed as a luxury that cannot be afforded, but as a viable alternative, hospices will continue to survive and increase in number.

NOTES

[1] Glen W. Davidson, "Five Models for Hospice Care," *Quality Review Bulletin,* May 1979, p. 8.

[2] *Ibid.,* p. 9.

[3] *Ibid.,* p. 8.

[4] *Loc. cit.*

[5] John A. Hackley, "Full-Service Hospice Offers, Home, Day, and Inpatient Care," *Hospitals,* November 1, 1977, p. 84.

[6] Claire F. Ryder and Diane M. Ross, "Terminal Care—Issues and Alternatives," *Public Health Reports* (92)1 (January-February 1977):26.

[7] Richard P. Ames, David Mineau, and Kathy Petrushevich, "Mercy Hospice: A Hospital-Based Program," *Hospital Progress,* March 1979, p. 63.

[8] Sr. Teresa Marie McIntier, "Hillhaven Hospice: A Freestanding, Family-Centered Program," *Hospital Progress,* March 1979, p. 68.

[9] *Blue Cross and Blue Shield of Michigan Hospice Program Pilot Project: Final Report,* Provider Pilot Programs Health Care Affairs, under the direction of Regina Weipert, November 15, 1983.

[10] Karen Rak, *Home Health Line* 9 (June 25, 1984):161.

[11] *Ibid.,* pp. 20, 131.

[12] *Ibid.,* p. 161.

[13] *Ibid.,* pp. 125, 131.

[14] Karen Rak, *Home Health Line* 8 (July 25, 1983):128; (August 1, 1983):128.

[15] Karen Rak, *Home Health Line* 8 (September 26, 1983):175.

[16] *Ibid.,* p. 179.

[17] *The National Hospice Reimbursement Act: How a Hospice and a Home Health Agency Can Structure Their Relationship to Meet the Core Service Requirement for Nursing Care.* NHO Monograph, Vienna, Va.: National Hospice Organization, 1983.

[18] *Ibid.,* p. 210.

[19] *Ibid.,* p. 206.

REFERENCES

Ames, Richard P., David Mineau, and Kathy Petrushevich. "Mercy Hospice: A Hospital-based Program." *Hospital Progress,* March 1979, pp. 63-67.

Davidson, Glen W. "Five Models for Hospice Care." *Quality Review Bulletin,* May 1979, pp. 8-9.

Ehrenfried, David, and Neil Hollander. "Reimbursing Hospice·Care: A Blue Cross and Blue Shield Perspective." *Hospital Progress,* March 1979, pp. 54-56.

Hackley, John A. "Full-Service Hospice Offers Home, Day and Inpatient Care." *Hospitals,* 51 (November 1, 1977):84-87.

"HCFA Medicare Program: Hospice Care." *Federal Register,* December 16, 1983.

McIntier, Sr. Teresa Marie, C.S.S. "Hillhaven Hospice: A Freestanding, Family-Centered Program." *Hospital Progress,* March 1979, pp. 68-72.

National Hospice Organization. *NHO Hospice Monograph: The National Hospice Reimbursement Act (1983).* Vienna, Va.: NHO, 1983.

National Hospice Organization. *NHO Hospice Monograph: The National Hospice Reimbursement Act (1984).* Vienna, Va.: NHO, 1983.

Ryder, Claire F., and Diane M. Ross. "Terminal Care—Issues and Alternatives." *Public Health Reports,* (92)1 (January-February 1977):20-29.

Spiegel, Allen D. *Home Healthcare.* Maryland: National Health Publishing, 1983.

Chapter 4

The Hospice Team

Myra J. Downs

Most discussions of hospice make the point that the care given to the hospice patient must be provided by an interdisciplinary team. The term "interdisciplinary team" implies more than just a group of professionals working with a patient. The team must consist of caring individuals who can communicate well with one another and support each other while using their individual knowledge and experience to benefit the patient and family. When these characteristics are present, the result is therapeutic care. This chapter will address the concept as well as the responsibilities of the interdisciplinary hospice team.

THE TEAM CONCEPT

The hospice team is the clinical component of any hospice program. It is an essential ingredient in the philosophy, management, and operation of hospice. The team members work together to identify and meet the needs of the hospice patient and family. The needs of a family facing the death of a loved one may be simple, requiring intervention by only a few members of the team, or complex, requiring at some time the work of all team members.

Traditionally the members of a hospice team have included nurses, home health aides, volunteers, social workers, nutritionists, pharmacists, psychologists, chaplains, speech/language pathologists, physical and occupational therapists, and the medical director. Members of other disciplines, such as dentists, are also finding a place on the hospice team. Anyone with a real interest and desire to both learn and teach can most likely be used on the team.

Qualifications of Team Members

All team members must have several qualities that enable them to function effectively in a group. First of all, they must be team players: they must be willing to share information and cooperate with the other team members. Second, they must be reliable, both for the patient's benefit and for the benefit of other team members. When they tell a family that they will come to the home at a certain time, they must meet that obligation. It is also important that all members attend team meetings regularly to serve as consultants to other team members. Third, hospice team members must have reached a personal understanding of death. They must be able to listen and share—mostly to listen—and provide a therapeutic atmosphere in which patients and families can express their feelings. And last and most important, team members must believe in hospice care. This will obviously enhance their effectiveness as well as their overall support of the program.

Special training for all team members is needed. The philosophy, goals and objectives, and particulars for the specific program in which the team is to function should be covered. Also, periodic continuing education programs should be provided for all team members. See Chapter 5 for detailed information on selection, training, and support of hospice workers.

TEAM COORDINATION

Rubin states that "if the basic mission or job requires that you and others must work together and coordinate your activities with each other, then you are a team."[1] The key word in this definition is *coordinate*. And coordination among members sometimes becomes difficult when various members of the team are volunteers who come into the hospice from different agencies. Therefore, careful planning and organization are essential for effective team functioning.

Weekly team meetings are an excellent medium for the exchange of ideas, problem solving, decision making, and overall coordination of the hospice team. If the team members must come from different areas, timing and location are important considerations. Often brown-bag lunch meetings or late afternoon meetings work best. If the hospice is contained within one agency or institution, early morning meetings may work well. It is most important to consider the specific needs of the team members in setting up the team meetings.

Team meetings should be organized and should follow an agenda. A sample agenda might include:

1. Review of minutes of the last meeting.

2. Presentation of new referrals.
3. Staffing needs of current patients.
4. Bereavement.

Information about each patient should be organized to provide each member with necessary information in a succinct manner. One useful method is the team conference worksheet (see Figure 4.1). This type of form provides updated information each week for the team and also allows space for notes on planning, discussion, and so forth that an individual team member may wish to document and keep. The worksheet is updated each week before the meeting by the team coordinator, who may be the nursing coordinator or another member of the team. Information is obtained from verbal reports and progress notes in the patient's records made by the various team members.

Minutes of team meetings should be kept in order to document team decisions. It is the team that makes the final decision regarding the admission of a patient, and the team record should document the reasons to admit or not admit for future reference. Often a volunteer can be found to attend team meetings and keep the minutes.

During team meetings much information is provided by members of different professional areas. This serves as an informal means of continuing education. For example, the speech pathologist might describe to the team the method of communication he has taught a patient who cannot speak. This sharing of information would aid the other members of the team in the delivery of holistic care to the patient and family and to future patients.

All members of the team may identify problems in the patient's home that need discussion. Through the specialized education and experience of the various team members, several possible solutions to complex problems may be identified that could be presented as alternatives to the patient and family. Important to note here is the fact that the patient and family are also part of the comprehensive team effort. Decisions about the patient's care are not made in isolation but rather in concert with the patient's desires and are always discussed with the patient and with the primary caregiver.

Team Support Group

Working daily with a hospice program can place tremendous stress on the team members. Effective stress management is essential to prevent conflict or burnout. The hospice team member functions in an environment that provides a ripe medium for the growth of stress. Regularly scheduled team support group meetings have been shown to be effective in reducing stress in many hospice programs. The leader should be

Figure 4.1. Team conference worksheet.

Date _____

Patient	Diagnosis/ Prognosis	Physician	Patient Problems	Nurse	Volunteer	Notes

someone with group work experience, preferably a psychologist or social worker. The purpose of the group is simply for everyone to talk about the problems he or she faces and therefore to work through the stressors that are present. Team members are encouraged to participate in the counseling sessions. (For more information, see Chapter 5.)

Record Keeping

A comprehensive medical record is necessary in a hospice program. The record should be well organized and should contain the appropriate forms required for JCAH accreditation or Medicare certification. All professional members of the team are required to make entries in the record documenting their activities and plan of care. Many programs have adopted the NLN Problem-Oriented Record System, which can be obtained from the NLN Publications Order Unit.

ROLE OF THE NURSE

The nurse often serves as the coordinator of the hospice team. This role suits the nurse well, as she usually has more contact with the patient than other team members and therefore can make frequent assessments of the patient's needs and capabilities. These assessments allow her to keep abreast of changes in the patient's situation and call other professionals into the home as needs are identified. The nurse who assumes the role of team coordinator must be aware of every means of technological assistance available that might help the patient. She must also be unselfish and must see herself as a part of a team: she must be willing to have other team members participate in the patient's care.

The nurse may also fill the role of clinician, giving direct patient care. The nurse has the body of theoretical and practical knowledge needed to provide care to hospice patients. For example, she is aware of measures that can be used for pain and symptom control in individual patients and what techniques work best for maintaining optimum nutritional intake and normal bowel functioning. Also, many hospice nurses have become certified in the administration of chemotherapy, which is sometimes used in palliative care. The role of nurse-clinician in hospice care is very broad, ranging from helping the patient with psychosocial needs to managing complex pain-control procedures.

A hospice nurse is on call 24 hours a day. It is usually agreed that it is not feasible for members of other disciplines to share the on-call responsibility as most of the needs that arise can best be addressed by the nurse. Adequate compensation, as well as a well-planned rotation schedule, are important aspects of the 24-hour on-call responsibility. Also, inherent in the nurse's clinican role is the supervision of other nursing support personnel in the home, such as home health aides and patient care volunteers. Care must be given to this nursing function so that optimum utilization of these personnel may be obtained and the patient and family may receive maximum benefits.

The nurse also serves as a consultant to other team members. Because she may see the patient more frequently than they do, the nurse can provide up-to-date information to the team, thus helping other team members make appropriate decisions about their plans of care. The information the nurse provides may also aid the volunteer director in assigning volunteers in the homes. Through her observations, the nurse may be able to determine which volunteers will be able to interact best with which patients.

The nurse's observation and judgment can also be important to program administration. Through day-to-day hospice nursing care delivery, the nurse may determine that there is a need for changes in current program policies or for the formulation of additional policies.

Consultant to the primary physician is an important aspect of the nurse's role. The primary physician relies on the nurse's accurate, comprehensive professional judgment to stay informed, and together the nurse, physician, and patient can make appropriate decisions to improve patient care and quality of life.

The hospice nurse also serves as an educator to the team, the patient and family, and the community. Hospice is not a well-understood concept in many areas of the country, and community-wide education is often needed. The hospice nurse is often the appropriate person to conduct seminars and make presentations to community groups. Also, the nurse may provide inservice educational programs to other team members on such topics as pain and symptom management or proper body mechanics. Inherent in team functioning is the blending of roles, and the nurse facilitates this by teaching other team members certain nursing procedures, which can contribute greatly to continuity of care.

The family members become students of the hospice nurse. She may teach them to feed or bathe the patient, give injections, or position him, as well as other procedures that support and provide comfort. In working with the caregivers the nurse must assess their learning readiness and not expect too much from them too soon. Remembering their stress level and working with them, reinforcing what they have been taught, and encouraging them will aid the nurse in teaching home care techniques to the family.

Job descriptions for a hospice nurse and for other team members appear at the end of this chapter. In addition, Chapter 6 provides an extensive discussion of the role of the hospice nurse-administrator and nurse-clinician.

ROLES OF OTHER TEAM MEMBERS

Chaplain

The hospice chaplain works with the family and the patient to provide support and helps them in meeting their spiritual needs. The chaplain may work directly with the patient and family or he may work with the family's own clergyman. If he does the latter, his role becomes that of a consultant; if he works directly with the patient and family he must be able to work with people of different faiths, providing for them an atmosphere in which they can express their doubts, fears, and beliefs. A minister who has received training as a hospital chaplain should have this ability.

The chaplain may also serve as a support person or consultant to other team members. The patient may choose to express his religious feelings to another member of the team, and the chaplain may need to provide information to that team member to enable him or her to be more effective. The chaplain should also keep the team informed about any specific desires or religious customs of the patient; this will increase continuity of care. In addition, the hospice chaplain should serve as a resource in the community to other clergymen, educating them about the hospice concept as well as about his specific role on the team.

Medical Social Worker

The role of the medical social worker in the hospice is broad and varied. The social worker's two most common roles are counselor for the patient and family and liaison with community agencies seeking resources to meet the patient's needs. Because the medical social worker has extensive training in the area of counseling, he can help the patient and family work through their feelings, both before the death and during the bereavement period. Although each person will respond to death and dying in his or her own unique way, all need support and understanding and the social worker is uniquely qualified to provide assistance in this area.

The social worker should be knowledgeable about all community resources and should provide all available information to other team members. Social workers are known for their creativity and ability to locate scarce resources when there is a need.

Speech/Language Pathologist

Communication is the heart of a hospice program, since an important goal of patients and families is to express their emotions. As a facilitator of communication, the speech/language pathologist can provide a valuable service to hospice patients and their families. When a patient no longer possesses the conventional method of communication—speech—other methods of communication can be found. Communication boards and sign language are two of the methods that can give the patient and family the ability to work together, share their feelings, and say things that might otherwise have had to go unsaid. A speech/language pathologist working directly with the patient and family as well as serving as a consultant to the team can enhance the quality of care hospice patients and their families receive.

Dentist

The dental needs of a hospice patient can best be met by a dentist who is familiar with the hospice concept. Ideally, the dentist should be an integral part of the interdisciplinary team. The nurse should include a dental evaluation in her initial assessment so the patient's needs can be discussed at team conferences and plans made for treatment. Often the dentist must care for the patient in the home, which may be difficult. However, the dental services rendered to the hospice patient are generally surgical or prosthodontic in nature, and these can usually be carried out adequately in the home.

There are several indications for dental treatment of a hospice patient, including (1) maintenance of self-image, (2) decreased masticatory function, (3) pain or infection, and (4) loose or ill-fitting dentures. One of the most important reasons for dental intervention is the maintenance of the patient's self-image, as this is an important goal in hospice care. Dental treatment can play an important role in either maintaining or restoring the patient's appearance.

Adequate masticatory function is vital to good nutrition. The dentist may work with the patient to remove the cause for the patient's inability to chew properly, and, working closely with other team members, may help the patient improve his nutritional status.

A common complaint of edentulous patients is loose-fitting dentures. The dentist has several modalities of treatment available that can correct this situation, again enhancing the patient's appearance and self-image and possibly improving his nutritional status.

Nutritionist

Since adequate nutrition is a goal for the hospice patient, the nutritionist is a valuable member of the team. Often as a disease progresses appetite and taste decrease, making maintenance of adequate nutrition difficult. The nutritionist can often provide the patient and family with information, ideas, or suggestions which can enhance the patient's dietary intake. Maintaining a high-protein, high-carbohydrate diet is often the goal, and food supplements as well as careful calculation of caloric intake may be necessary. The nutritionist attends team conferences and shares information with other team members to enable them to help the patient and family meet the nutritional goals.

The nutritionist works closely with family members to determine goals for the patient and find realistic ways to reach these goals. Often the method of food preparation or the frequency of meals requires changing. Maintenance of adequate nutritional intake not only helps the patient but also provides a source of comfort to the family, who feel they are contributing to making the patient more comfortable.

Occupational Therapist

With good nursing and medical care, pain and symptoms associated with terminal illness can often be abated within a few days, without addiction or detrimental side effects. It is then, however, that real problems of living may arise, and it is at this point that the occupational therapist's skills may be necessary. Once the patient's symptoms are controlled, he may begin worrying about the future: the patient needs to work at something useful and relevant to him in order to improve his morale. The experienced occupational therapist can provide work for the patient that will aid in restoring his dignity and help give meaning to life regardless of the amount of time left to the patient.

Physical Therapist

Serving as a member of the interdisciplinary team, the physical therapist can provide a valuable service to team members as well as to the patient and family. The physical therapist's goals for a hospice patient may be different than for other patients; however, restoration to a maximum level of functioning, increasing or preserving some degree of independence, and teaching family members or volunteers such procedures as transfer techniques, are all worthwhile goals of physical therapy for hospice patients. A physical therapist will not be needed on each hospice case; however, the physical therapist can often help patients live as comfortably and richly as possible.

Pharmacist

Pain management and symptom control are usually considered nursing and medicine's responsibility; however, a pharmacist can provide valuable assistance in these areas. Serving in the role of consultant to the team, the pharmacist can discuss drug action and interaction as well as give advice on specific regimes based on a patient's individual problems. He may also advise the team about particular side effects of certain drugs and provide information on how to alleviate these side effects.

Home Health Aide

The nursing or home health aide serves as a valuable member of the team. She often becomes very close to the patient, as she usually spends a great deal of time with him giving personal care. The aide may be able to discover a potential problem early, such as a reddened area on a bony prominence, and give information to the nurse so that additional preventive measures can be undertaken. The aide and nurse must work closely together in order to provide the most comprehensive care possible. Aides should be included in team conferences and their contributions should be encouraged.

Psychologist

The ultimate goal for the hospice caregiver is to bring about peaceful acceptance of death or at least to provide an opportunity for the patient to relate his feelings.[2] Through direct intervention or consultation with other team members, the psychologist can be instrumental in meeting this goal. He should be able to teach the team methods of therapeutic communication. Intense feelings can be frightening, and the psychologist can help the team members work through these feelings so that they can provide support to the patient and family.

Medical Director

The hospice medical director serves as a consultant to the team, the primary physician, and the overall medical community. He must be qualified to respond to the needs of the terminally ill patient as well as to serve as an advocate for the hospice concept. He should be available to attend team meetings and should stay informed about the condition of all the hospice patients. In some situations he may be called on to serve as a liaison between the hospice team and the primary physician. In no cases should the medical director be expected to take medical responsibility for a hospice patient unless he is also the primary physician. By providing information about disease processes, medical regimes, and so forth, the medical director enables the team to deliver better care.

SUMMARY

The focus of care in hospice is the patient and family, and care is delivered by an interdisciplinary team. Frequent team meetings are held to allow for interaction of the team members. Through this collaborative process, the diverse needs of patients and their families are systematically analyzed and plans of action are proposed to provide therapeutic and supportive care. The unique contributions of each team member create a synergistic forum that not only enhances the quality of care but also provides for the individual growth and development of the team members.

NOTES

[1] F. Rubin et.al., *Improving the Coordination of Care: A Program for Health Team Development*. Cambridge, Mass.: Ballinger, 1975.

[2] Patricia E. Greene, "The Pivotal Role of the Nurse in Hospice Care," *Ca—A Cancer Journal for Clinicians*, July/August, 1984, p. 204.

REFERENCES

Betros, Cecil, and Myra Downs. "The Role of the Speech/Language Pathologist in Hospice." *The Journal of the American Speech – Language – Hearing Association*, June 1984, p. 302.

Cerino, Noreen D. "Therapeutic Communication: A Necessity in Hospice Care." *The American Journal of Hospice Care*, Spring 1984, p. 21.

Greene, Patricia E. "The Pivotal Role of the Nurse in Hospice Care," *Ca—A Cancer Journal for Clinicians*, July/August 1984, p. 204.

Picard, Helen B., and Josefina B. Magno. "The Role of Occupational Therapy in Hospice Care." *The American Journal of Occupational Therapy*, September 1982, p. 597.

JOB DESCRIPTION: HOSPICE NURSE

Definition

This is a responsible professional nurse position that requires clinical skills and experience in working with terminally ill patients and their families in the home. It also requires interpersonal skills that permit services to be provided through an interdisciplinary team approach.

Examples of Duties

Makes home visits, assesses the family's needs, and makes appropriate suggestions for referrals to the hospice nurse coordinator.

Presents cases in team conference and elicits recommendations from team members regarding how the patient's and family's needs may be met using the holistic approach of the interdisciplinary hospice team.

Assists hospice nurse coordinator in preparing physician's orders to guide skilled activities that are consistent with the attending physician's plan of care and based on documented patient and family assessments.

Develops a trusting relationship with the patient and family.

Observes clinical signs and symptoms; reports to hospice nurse coordinator reactions to treatment, including drugs, and changes in the patient's physical and emotional condition.

Collects blood samples or other diagnostic specimens to be sent to the laboratory for monitoring the patient's treatment and care.

Informs both physician and team of changes and development in the patient's or family's condition.

Teaches, supervises, and counsels the patient and family members regarding the nursing needs and other related problems of the terminally ill in the home (medication administration, pain control, symptom control, side effects, etc.).

Gives personal care to patient as needed.

Supervises the patient care activity of the home health aide and the family's private-duty caregivers, registered nurses, licensed practical nurses, and sitters.

Shares on-call service 24 hours per day with hospice nurse coordinator.

Participates in bereavement follow-up.

Seeks continuing education opportunities to provide for professional growth.

Assists with the orientation of new hospice nurses as assigned by the supervisor.

Minimum Qualifications

Required knowledge, skills, and abilities: Must be licensed to practice nursing in the state and be skilled in the areas of physical assessment, patient assessment, and family assessment.

Education: Bachelor's degree in nursing preferred.

Experience: Home care experience desired. Must have practiced as an RN for a minimum of two years.

JOB DESCRIPTION: HOSPICE NURSE COORDINATOR

Definition

This professional requires leadership and organizational skills and interpersonal skills that permit services to be provided through an interdisciplinary team approach. The coordinator leads and manages development of the hospice program and oversees day-to-day functioning of the hospice. Responsible for the overall planning, delivery, and evaluation of quality nursing care for hospice patients and their families. Instructs, supervises, and evaluates nursing personnel and volunteers. Coordinates services of all team members. Directs admission of patients to hospice program.

Examples of Duties

Coordinates the development of hospice policies and procedures.

Initiates policy and program evaluation based on research findings, current trends, and needs of county hospice organization.

Provides leadership and coordination of team efforts as needed.

Assists in the preparation of yearly budgets for the hospice program.

Coordinates orientation and inservice programs for the hospice team and volunteers on an ongoing basis.

Collaborates with other agencies and professional groups to promote the hospice concept in the community.

Provides a monthly report of hospice progress to the chairman of professional advisory board.

Facilitates weekly interdisciplinary team meetings.

Evaluates the effectiveness of services provided through utilization review, chart audit, monthly reports, and other methods.

Facilitates communication between the hospice team and the primary physician during the patient's course of service.

Provides on-call service 24 hours per day, supplemented by hospice nurse volunteers.

Coordinates meetings and efforts of the hospice professional advisory board.

Represents the hospice program with outside organizations and institutions.

Coordinates the discharge of patients and families from the hospice program.

Assists with publicity and public relations.

Serves on the hospice professional advisory board.

Administers chemotherapy to hospice patients as required.

Maintains records for the hospice volunteer program.

Assists with fund-raising efforts.

Maintains effective collaboration and liaison with hospice medical director.

Develops community education programs in hospice care in concert with hospice team and volunteers.

Oversees development and maintenance of records related to hospice care in accordance with requirements of Joint Commission.

Works with medical director in maintaining close relationships with medical staff.

Consults with potential patients and families and facilitates their admission.

Attends meetings as necessary.

Delivers or supervises delivery of home care education of primary caregiver before patient's discharge from hospital.

Coordinates activities of all team members and volunteers in homes.

Contributes to education of other professionals by means of lectures, written materials, and observation in hospice. Attends various meetings to enhance skills in hospice care and management.

Plans and implements hospice quality assurance program in cooperation with the professional standards committee.

Visits patients and families periodically in homes to evaluate needs and assess effectiveness of hospice team and volunteers.

Provides direct care to patients and their families when specialized skills are needed.

Acts as patient advocate.

Maintains effective liaison with department heads who furnish personnel and services to hospice program, e.g., director of physical therapy, social services.

Maintains schedules for vacations, on-call hours, and days off for all hospice staff and volunteers.

Evaluates performance of each nurse on a regular basis and provides appropriate feedback.

Reporting Relationship

Reports to the vice-president.

Education

BS degree in nursing. Must be licensed as a Registered Nurse. Must be certified in chemotherapy administration.

Required Knowledge, Skills, and Abilities

Ability to organize and coordinate an interdisciplinary team; ability to speak in public and present a positive image of the hospice program; ability to assess the scope and effectiveness of services provided by the hospice program.

JOB DESCRIPTION: NUTRITIONIST

Definition

Provides nutritional counseling to patients and families, as well as consultation to the hospice interdisciplinary team.

Examples of Duties

Provides nutritional counseling and assessment as indicated for patients and families.

Makes home visits as required by hospice nurse coordinator.

Serves as a member of the hospice interdisciplinary team.

Provides inservice education to the hospice interdisciplinary team.

Provides consultation to team members and volunteers as needed.

Minimum Qualifications

Education: Must have a bachelor of science degree and be a registered dietitian (RD).

Experience: Two years' experience, with hospital or community health experience preferred.

JOB DESCRIPTION: PHARMACIST

Definition

This professional provides consultation and education to members of the hospice interdisciplinary team.

Examples of Duties

Serves as a member of the hospice interdisciplinary team.

Provides drug information to hospice team members, referring physicians, patients, and families as indicated.

Provides inservice education to the hospice team.

Minimum Qualifications

Education: Minimum of bachelor of science in pharmacy.

Experience: Minimum of three years' pharmaceutical experience.

JOB DESCRIPTION: PHYSICAL THERAPIST

Definition

Identifies and provides for physical therapy of patients and families. Coordinates efforts with those of other hospice team members.

Examples of Duties

Initiates contact with patient at the request of the hospice nurse coordinator.

Evaluates patients' physical therapy needs and provides treatment to patients as well as instructions to patients and families.

Provides inservice education to hospice team and volunteers.

Serves as a member of the hospice interdisciplinary team.

Minimum Qualifications

Education: Bachelor of science degree in physical therapy and a current state license to practice physical therapy.

Experience: Two years' experience as a physical therapist with experience in home health care preferred.

JOB DESCRIPTION: HOSPICE CHAPLAIN

Definition

This professional provides spiritual counseling, consultation, and education to patients, families, and interdisciplinary team members.

Examples of Duties

Serves as a member of the hospice interdisciplinary team.

Coordinates with area clergymen the spiritual care of patients and families.

Provides pastoral support to the hospice team.

Serves as a pastoral caregiver to selected patients and families.

Provides inservice education to the hospice interdisciplinary team as well as to community pastors.

Minimum Qualifications

Experience: Three years of local church pastoral experience or its equivalent.

JOB DESCRIPTION: DIRECTOR OF VOLUNTEERS

Definition

Recruits, trains, and screens volunteers for hospice program. Maintains record of name, address, phone number, and type of service of active volunteers.

Examples of Duties

Contributes as a team member at interdisciplinary team meetings.

Interviews, trains, and assesses prospective volunteers.

Attends monthly professional advisory board meetings.

Conducts annual evaluations with each volunteer in conjunction with nurse coordinator.

Initiates volunteer staff development on a quarterly basis or more often as needed.

Conducts ongoing evaluation of the volunteer program.

Reporting Relationship

Reports to nurse coordinator.

JOB DESCRIPTION: SUPPORT-GROUP LEADER

Definition

This professional provides leadership for the support group for hospice team members and volunteers. He or she provides consultation, training, and education to the team members and volunteers to enable them to deal with the emotional and psychological components of terminal illness.

Examples of Duties

Serves as a member of the hospice interdisciplinary team.

Provides training in communication skills for hospice volunteers and team members.

Provides training and consultation to hospice volunteers and team members in working with patients and families experiencing grief reactions.

Serves as support-group leader for emotional support for hospice volunteers and team members, providing group and individual counseling as needed.

Minimum Qualifications

Education: Master's degree in psychology.

Experience: Three years' postgraduate experience in working in a psychological setting. Experience in working with terminally ill patients preferred.

JOB DESCRIPTION: SPEECH/LANGUAGE PATHOLOGIST

Definition

Identifies and provides for communication needs of patients and families. Coordinates activities with those of other hospice team members and provides consultation services to interdisciplinary team.

Examples of Duties

Initiates contact with patient at the request of the hospice nurse coordinator.

Evaluates patients' and families' communication needs; provides treatment to patients and instruction to patient and family.

Serves as a consultant to team members on developing alternative communication systems for patients; instructs team members in different approaches for enhancing communication.

Minimum Qualifications

Education: Master of science degree in speech/language pathology. Certified by American Speech/Language-Hearing Association. Current license to practice speech/language pathology.

Experience: Two years' experience beyond the clinical fellowship year, with experience in home health care preferred.

JOB DESCRIPTION: MEDICAL DIRECTOR

Definition

Provides medical information and consultation to hospice team members, community physicians, patients, and families.

Examples of Duties

Consults, upon request, with attending physicians regarding pain and symptom management.

In the absence of the attending physician, provides consultation and medical information to hospice team members.

Serves as a medical liaison with community physicians.

Determines patient medical eligibility for the hospice program in accordance with hospice policies.

Serves as a member of the hospice team.

Coordinates effort with community physicians to provide care in the event the primary physician is unable to retain responsibility for patient care.

Provides inservice education to the hospice team members as needed.

Minimum Qualifications

Education: Licensed as a physician. Medical oncology specialization preferred.

JOB DESCRIPTION: HOME HEALTH AIDE/ HOMEMAKER VOLUNTEER

Definition

The home health aide/homemaker volunteer provides direct patient care in the home. Services are supervised by a registered nurse. Duties may include giving patient care, ambulating patients, using proper transfer techniques, preparing light meals, or doing minor housekeeping tasks. Home health aides/homemaker volunteers also provide housekeeping services to individuals who, because of infirmity or disability, could not remain in their own homes without them.

Examples of Duties

Assists the patients with activities of daily living, which may include bathing, giving oral hygiene, caring for nails, shampooing, or shaving.

Uses safe transfer techniques when transferring a patient from the bed to a wheelchair or other assistive devices.

Helps patients to ambulate as directed by their physicians.

Assists patients with simple exercises under the supervision of the home care nurse or physical therapist.

Changes an occupied bed, using proper body positioning.

Performs incidental household services that are essential for the patient's well-being in the home.

Reports improvements or unusual changes pertinent to the patient's care in the home to the home care nurse or nurse coordinator.

Assists with personal care such as baths and shampoos.

Performs light housekeeping duties, but does not do seasonal housecleaning.

Buys groceries and other household items as indicated.

Does the patient's light laundry, but no heavy family laundry.

Assists the patient in following the doctor's treatment plan by encouraging the proper use of assistive devices.

Demonstrates, by examples, better homemaking for the culturally or economically deprived individual.

Records daily home care visits in an appropriate manner on the patient's record.

Completes a daily encounter sheet of daily activities.

Keeps an accurate mileage record.

Performs related duties as indicated.

Required Knowledge, Skills, and Abilities

Current driver's license. High school graduate or a GED equivalency.

Chapter 5

Staffing and Stress Management

Barbara M. Petrosino

No program of care can make having terminal cancer pleasant, nor can it make death easy for the patient and the family. Hospice is no exception. Photos of dying patients who are smiling and relaxed are a source of satisfaction to those involved in patient care, but these pictures can be frustrating to staff members and families when other patients' serious and complex problems do not allow for such ideal results. Selecting staff members and helping them deal with stress are therefore important factors in a successful hospice program. This chapter discusses the hospice administrator's role in staffing and stress management.

CRITERIA FOR STAFF SELECTION

A smooth-running, efficient hospice organization is due in large part to careful and deliberate staff selection. Obtaining the right mix of workers who can both work together smoothly as a team and function effectively as individuals is a must. Therefore, when hiring new staff members, the hospice administrator must first assess the personal and professional characteristics of the existing staff members and the needs of the organization. Criteria derived for persons needed to fill vacancies should include attributes that will complement the abilities of the current staff.

Motivation

Prospective staff members' motivation for wanting to work with terminally ill patients is an important factor to consider. Healthy motivation is composed of both desire to do the work and an objective assessment of one's abilities. Desire in this context means wanting to use one's abilities to achieve the stated goal of hospice care, to improve the quality of the patient's remaining life through pain relief and comfort measures. Necessary abilities for a potential hospice nurse include clinical skills in both the psychomotor and interpersonal realms, as well as sound clinical judgment.

Vachon cautions against hiring individuals who enter hospice work with strong personal needs, which later surface and cause stress within the organization.[1] She suggests that inappropriate motivators for hospice work may include a desire to be involved in a popular cause; to follow a respected acquaintance; to be free of the policies of inpatient facilities; to have more convenient work hours; to control or master death and the illness and pain associated with it; to act out a religious or humanistic "calling"; or to work through an unresolved personal experience. While some aspects of these motivators are present in many competent employees, they are generally unhealthy as primary motivators and may become sources of stress in the employee's future interactions with staff as well as with families and patients.

Other Characteristics

There are some general personality characteristics that are essential to an effective and productive hospice staff. Hospice staff members need to be flexible: they must be able to move comfortably from conventional methods to creative and innovative solutions to problems. They must also be sensitive to the unstated needs of patients and families as well as of fellow staff members. They must be professionally competent. Most important, they must bring a maturity, not necessarily of age, but of life experience and personal philosophy, to the position. A list of desirable personal characteristics for hospice staff has been developed by personnel from The Hospice of Marin. A modified version of this listing follows:[2]

- Assertiveness.
- High level of personal energy.
- Self-awareness; willingness to probe motivations, openness to learning, growing, and changing.
- Sensitivity to others.
- Ability to function without traditional role constraints.

Ability to function under stress.

Ability to make decisions alone and accept responsibility for them.

Ability to set limits.

Ability to be in touch with feelings.

Equal ability to deal with physical and emotional components of patient's needs.

Able to "be," not necessarily to "do."

Ability to acccept a challenge.

Ability to act independently yet function effectively within a group.

It is unlikely that any job applicant will possess all of these characteristics; therefore, the administrator must set priorities and consider compromises. It is possible that an applicant without all of the desired characteristics may have the potential and interest to develop them. Hiring someone is always a gamble, but the administrator who objectively thinks through the agency's needs and gathers as much information as possible reduces the risks involved. There are very few organizations that have not made serious hiring errors. Correction of the error before staff functioning is disrupted is a mark of an effective administrator.

APPLICATIONS AND INTERVIEWS

The employment application should include routine information (age, sex, education, work history, licensure status). In addition, it should include specific questions directed toward eliciting information about the candidate's life experiences, work experiences, interpersonal relationships, experiences with death, and other stressful events. The questions should require narrative answers in which the candidate carries out some self-examination. Both the application itself and the interview format must avoid questions that can be interpreted as being discriminatory. Only information that relates directly to the candidate's qualifications for the job can be legally sought in this country. The Equal Employment Opportunities Commission can provide guidelines and restrictions.

The names of professional and personal references should be requested of all candidates. Telephone contacts with the references are recommended, because more information can generally be acquired verbally than through the mail. Careful inquiry should be made about the candidate's interpersonal relations, teamwork, professional competence, and performance under stress. (A format for an effective telephone inquiry is presented by Mount.[3])

Candidates whose applications show promise should be invited for interviews. The interview should provide an opportunity for the administrator to learn more about the applicant as well as for the applicant to find out about the hospice and the specific job. The administrator should provide a broad description of the hospice concept and the philosophy and characteristics of the specific hospice. Job requirements and employment benefits should be specifically described.

During the interview the administrator should attempt to verify information provided on the application and obtained from the references. Further information should also be elicited about the applicant's motivation for working with the dying, general religious or spiritual beliefs, personality characteristics, professional goals, and personal strengths and weaknesses. Broad, open-ended questions that allow the applicant to do most of the talking can reveal a great deal of information.

It may also be helpful for a staff member of the applicant's discipline to speak with the applicant to provide further information and to help evaluate professional competence. The staff person can describe the agency's day-to-day operations and can perhaps arrange for the applicant to accompany a nurse on a home visit. This interaction between staff member and applicant also involves staff members in organizational decision making.

LaGrand[4] provides the following guidelines for eliciting useful information in an interview:

> **Motivation to Serve Others:** Is the candidate overly committed with few outside interests or are convenience and remunerative considerations of the highest priority? Why has the individual applied for the job? Careful assessment of the reasons for a person's interest in hospice work can uncover factors indicating stability or instability when confronting job stress. A key indicator is the awareness of one's limits.
>
> **Personality Characteristics and Job Compatibility:** Does the candidate need to be in complete control of the job to the extent that the belief exists that the job cannot be accomplished by someone else? Can the candidate share responsibilities? Are there signs of a sense of humor? Humor can often be a resource in coping with stressing interpersonal relationships. Conversely, the all-too-dedicated, staid, and serious may themselves add to, rather than manage, the unexpected contingency.
>
> **Ability to Relate to Others:** Skills in self-disclosure, building trust, and adjusting to rapidly changing circumstances are most desirable and helpful in stress management. Are loyalty and compassion part of the candidate's ability to relate? Are there indications the

candidate would socialize appropriately with other staff members outside of the work setting?

Handling High-Stress Situations: Has past work experience given evidence of meeting duress and coping with the unexpected? What does the candidate do to manage the stresses of his or her particular lifestyle? What is the nature of the candidate's outside interests? Are there hobbies or recreational pursuits?

Work Goals: People can be fully committed to fitting into the organization or team and yet have goals which cannot possibly be met in a particular work setting. Interviews must probe the job expectations of the candidate and his or her willingness to try different approaches as dictated by the job description. Also the specific goals of the employing organization must be spelled out to the candidate and reactions must be sought to assess compatibility.

Physical Condition, Vitality, and Energy Levels: Service to the dying is both physically and emotionally demanding. Health and work records are important in determining illness patterns. If records are not available, inquiries should be made to obtain some indication of how frequently the candidate has been ill with colds, flu and other diseases. Sickness not only affects stress levels, but with some people, may be a reaction to on-the-job stress.

The goal of the interview should be to find the right person for the job, not to sell the hospice position to the candidate. Securing an employee under pressure may lead to unrealistic expectations on the part of the applicant and increased stress later on. Mount suggests that hiring decisions are too often made too quickly, either after interviewing an insufficient number of applicants or on the basis of superficial first impressions of the candidate.[5]

ORIENTATION

Preparing new employees to function effectively is an important part of staffing a hospice. A strong orientation program is an essential component of that preparation. The form of the orientation program for new hospice staff members varies from organization to organization. Lectures, simulations, role playing, videotapes, audiotapes, films, home visits, and prepackaged skills programs may be included. Many organizations use their own in-house orientation programs, while others combine training programs set up by other hospices. Attendance at professional conferences on terminal care, learning through supervised experience with hospice patients and families, and taking courses in related fields (e.g., counseling) can all be a part of an orientation program. The selection of activities should, in any case, meet the individual employee's specific learning needs.

The general topics commonly included in a hospice staff orientation are death and dying, the hospice concept, team functioning, individual roles of team members, policies and procedures of the organization, details of terminal care including legal requirements, family functioning, and pain and symptom control. Although courses in death and dying are now commonly included in professional education curricula, it is generally a mistake to assume that health professionals have sufficient background in meeting the complex psychosocial needs of terminally ill patients and their families. Palliative care (pain and symptom control), which is unique to hospice care, should also be a primary as well as ongoing focus of staff development for nurses. Most hospices collect articles, books, reprints, journals, newsletters, and research reports related to hospice care for further inservice education for staff members.

A vital component of the new employee's orientation is spending at least a week or two "shadowing" an experienced staff member. This gives the employee an opportunity to (1) visit patients and families and then discuss their needs and approaches for meeting them; (2) observe office procedures and review policies and patient record systems in detail; (3) attend team conferences to learn about both their process and content; and (4) observe institutional interrelationships, the use of community resources, the use of volunteers, and the bereavement program and thus become more familiar with the overall organization.

This framework should enable new employees to identify their own strengths and weaknesses and needs for further training. A thorough, well-planned orientation and training program can be an important means of preventing staff stress. The program should provide a realistic picture of what can be accomplished with terminally ill patients and their families. The recognition that not all patients "die at peace, with their loving family at their side and their dog on the bed" is essential.

All new employees should be on probation for a well-defined period, usually 4, 6, or 12 weeks. At the end of this period, the employee and supervisor should mutually evaluate the employee's performance, in order to answer the question, "Is this the right match of person and position at this time?" In this way, both parties have the opportunity to suggest continuation or noncontinuation of employment. It is important to allow the employee an opportunity to say, "This is not for me at this time." It is also important for the employer to be able to terminate the relationship in the same way. This approach can also be used at other stages in a person's employment during regular evaluation sessions. It is important for an employee to leave not with a sense of failure but rather with the feeling that "I cannot do this work at this time."

STAFFING NEEDS

Personnel requirements for hospices vary greatly, depending on factors such as the stage of development of the organization, type of facility, geographic area covered, rural or urban location, available community resources, and economic and ethnic groups served. The appropriate standard of measurement, however, should be whether there are sufficient numbers of staff members to provide complete services to the patients and families accepted for care.

The developmental stage of a hospice influences staffing needs. A new hospice generally requires proportionately more staff members per patient served than an established one, because a greater amount of time is consumed in establishing procedures, refining mechanical operations such as recording and reporting, and establishing community relationships. A well-established organization can provide care for more patients with the same size staff. As staff members become more experienced and sophisticated, they can usually work more quickly and more effectively.

The type of facility especially influences the need for nursing staff. Inpatient facilities require larger professional nursing staffs. The staff is responsible for 24-hour care and frequently is called upon to provide more complex care than is done in the home. Home-care staff provide less direct care themselves and spend more time teaching, supervising, and providing support for the primary caregivers.

The size of the geographic area served is especially significant for home-care hospices because of the amount of time it takes staff members to travel from one home to another. With large amounts of travel time, staff members can make fewer visits each day.

The location of the hospice—urban versus rural—also influences staffing needs. An urban hospice generally has more well-established support services available to it, and therefore staff members can easily make referrals. Staff members in rural hospices frequently must provide more services themselves or spend more time training and coordinating volunteers to carry out support services (e.g., homemakers, transportation, diversional therapies).

In hospices with primarily poor patients, staff members must spend a great deal of time finding financial resources. Generally, more affluent patients qualify for more third-party reimbursement of services, or they have private means to pay for services. The more time staff members spend on indirect services to patients (i.e., economic), the fewer patients they are able to see each day.

Members of some ethnic groups have a strong family orientation. Therefore an extensive support system is already in place for the patient and caregivers are readily identifiable and available. Conversely, if the clientele is primarily composed of persons who have small families or no available family members, the staff may become involved in extensive coordination to secure adequate caregivers.

Some general guidelines for personnel requirements for both inpatient and home hospices and sample staffing patterns are presented in Table 5.1.[6] In determining the staffing needs of a particular organization, one must consider the factors previously discussed as well as these general guidelines.

TABLE 5.1
COMPARATIVE STAFFING FOR HOSPICES OF DIFFERENT TYPES AND SIZES

Staff Member*	Inpatient 6 Beds	Home Care 15 Patients	Home Care 30 Patients
Physician	.50	.25	.50
Head nurse	1	—	—
Home-care coordinator	—	—	1
Registered nurse (FTE)	5	3	3
Licensed vocational nurse (FTE)	2	—	—
Orderly	1	—	—
Nurse's aide	—	1	—
Home health aide	—	—	2
Ward clerk	1	—	—
Social worker	.50	.50	.50
Physiotherapist	.25	.25	.50
Pharmacist	.10	.10	.10
Recreational/music/ occupational therapist	.20	.20	.20
Dietitian/nutritionist	.10	.10	.10
Chaplain	.35	.50	.50
Volunteer coordinator	.50	.50	.50
Patient care volunteers (FTE)	3	2	3
Staff support person (psychiatrist/counselor/ psychologist)	.10	.10	.10

*Excluding medical director and administrative staff.

Source: ELM Services, Inc., "Workshop on Hospice Planning, Administration and Financing," Tucson, AZ, June 2-7, 1979.

SCHEDULING

Approaches to scheduling vary with the type of hospice and the viewpoints of the persons involved. The arrangement that results in the most effective patient care with the least stress for the staff is usually preferable.

Inpatient Units

Scheduling for the nursing staff of an inpatient hospice unit is similar to that in an acute-care hospital. Other staff members, such as the social worker, physical therapist, and occupational therapist, may vary their hours in an inpatient unit to meet patient needs. Many inpatient units follow the lead of London's St. Christopher's Hospice in designating a "family day off." Families are encouraged not to visit on these days except if the patient is in the immediate terminal stages. This permits families to take care of other responsibilities without a sense of guilt. Additional staff members may be scheduled to provide for patient care on family day off.

Home Care Programs

A variety of assignment patterns are common in home care programs. In some programs, the home-care coordinator may do all the intake assessments and then the patients are assigned to a primary nurse. This arrangement allows the home-care coordinator, who may not carry a caseload, to be familiar with all patients. Other programs rotate intake assessments among staff nurses for a specific time period. The nurse then may continue care of the patients she initially assessed.

In programs that cover large geographic areas, a team composed of a nurse, home health aide, and social worker may be assigned to a district or section of a city. Whenever possible, patient assignments should attempt to balance the complexity of care required, the stage of terminality, and the emotional state of the family. This attempt to plan the caseload can be helpful in reducing work-related stress as well as in reducing travel time.

In large hospice programs that include both inpatient and home care services, the staffs may be totally separate. This arrangement should not, however, preclude orientation assignments for all staff members in both settings, or even rotations to the other area on request.

On-Call Assignments

The primary care concept, with nurses taking calls from their own patients on a 24-hour basis, is not widely practiced because of the increased stress nurses experience as a result of never being off duty. Several different on-call patterns are possible: for example, nurses may take calls on a rotating basis of several days or a week at a time, with rotating weekends. This pattern allows the patient and family to become familiar with all staff members. Another arrangement is to employ a nurse or nurses exclusively for the on-call assignment and relieve the day staff of any on-call responsibility. In any hospice it is essential that all staff members trust the competence of all other staff members. Staff members must be able to relinquish total responsibility for a patient. This avoids fostering family dependence on any one staff member.

A careful introduction of the patient and the family to all the team members who may visit is important to the family's sense of security. The Hospice of Marin provides each family with a group picture of the staff.

Anticipatory teaching and guidance of the family during daily visits can significantly reduce the number of evening and night calls. The call nurse can further reduce the number of calls by establishing phone contact in the evening with certain families for reassurance and to discuss plans for the night. Often a reassuring conversation with the call nurse is all the family needs. A large number of calls is to be expected from the new patient and family until they are reassured that there is indeed someone available to talk to them.

Regardless of the patterns of assignment used, the hospice administrator must be sensitive to any staff member's need for relief: a day off, or assistance with an especially draining patient. Additional information about stress reduction appears later in this chapter.

SOURCES OF STRESS

Stress is an inevitable and healthful part of living. However, excessive stress is thought to contribute to dysfunctional behaviors and illness. Health care providers in areas such as intensive care, coronary care, oncology units, and emergency rooms are believed to experience high degrees of stress. Persons who consistently provide care for the terminally ill, and hospice personnel particularly, are also exposed to situations that produce high levels of stress. This section will explore some organizational, professional, and personal sources of stress for hospice workers, especially nurses.

Hospice Care as a Stressor

The nature of hospice care itself is a stressor for most caregivers. Continual exposure to dying patients and their emotionally distressed families creates great demands on the nurse, who often must deal with the patient's deteriorating physical and mental functioning while attempting to support grieving family members. As patients and their families move through the stages of dying, the nurse must handle their varying emotional responses (e.g., anger, fear, anxiety, remorse, guilt). Often the most important help the nurse can give is simply to share the difficult experience with the patient and the family. Sharing, however, requires a tremendous investment of self and is extremely draining for the nurse, for in the process, the finiteness of her life and the inevitability of her death surface and must be faced. The concurrent need to focus intensely on the needs of others and consider one's own needs can be a major stressor.

While some stress in caring for the dying is inevitable, certain situations are particular sources of stress for the hospice nurse. For example, a sudden death or the death of a patient before much has been done for him is usually very difficult. The death of a favorite patient or of a patient with whom the nurse has particularly identified (e.g., same sex, similar age or ethnic or socioeconomic background) can be unusually stressful. For most persons the death of a child or adolescent is particularly hard to accept. Nurses are no exception. Several deaths that occur in a short time period, or a long-drawn-out death, or the death of a person to whom a promise couldn't be kept (e.g., dying at home), or a death where the patient's family is unsatisfied with the care can all be sources of intensified stress for the nurse.

The fact that the concept of hospice care is different from other means of health care delivery can also serve as a stressor. Focusing on supportive and not curative goals is a philosophy different from that which most health caregivers, including nurses, internalized during their professional education. Frequently in hospice care the expressive role of nursing is emphasized more than the instrumental role. For example, sitting with the primary caregiver and discussing his concerns may be more appreciated than changing the patient's dressing. This reversal of emphasis is respected and welcomed by some nurses and is met by skepticism and avoidance by others. Most people, including nurses, have a strong need for peer approval. Involvement in something new can be exciting, but it can also be threatening.

Increased professional decision making and involvement as an integral part of an interdisciplinary team are ideas that have been emphasized in nursing education for many years. Implementation of these ideas has, however, been very slow in coming, and therefore many nurses have actually had very little experience in assuming significant responsibility for decision making in overall patient care or in extensive team participation. For example, hospice nurses are frequently expected to make recommendations to the physician about the types of medication needed. Adjustment of dosages and frequency of administration are often determined by the nurse based on her assessment of the patient's situation.

Decisions about admitting the patient to an inpatient facility are usually made by the nurse in conjunction with the patient, family, and physician. Nurses are expected to make substantive contributions in team conferences. More occasions for decision making and participation mean more occasions for making mistakes in judgments and for exposing oneself. Some nurses do not approve of or wish to assume these greater responsibilities. Thus to hospice nurses both the new activities and the lack of universal support from other nurses can be sources of additional stress.

Home care and on-call care are also frequent sources of stress for hospice nurses. Being available for calls around the clock can make the nurse feel tense or apprehensive. It can also create adjustment problems in the nurse's personal life.

Providing care in the home means being in the patient's or family's territory; the nurse is in effect an invited guest. The subtle difference in her degree of control over the situation can become a significant stressor, especially for the nurse who is accustomed to practicing in an inpatient facility.

Home care can also be stressful for nurses because of the absence of backup support facilities and personnel immediately accessible in inpatient facilities (e.g., peers, supervisors, physicians, and laboratory, dietary, respiratory, and physical therapy services). Home-care nurses often must fill a variety of roles, and they often feel like they are trying to be all things to all people. In the home, the nurse is frequently the only person with professional knowledge of pathology and symptomatology, and therefore the family often asks her about the cause of various symptoms and about the pathology of the patient's illness. The family usually wants immediate responses, and the nurse may or may not have the answers. In their attempt to schedule their lives around the patient, family members frequently ask unanswerable questions of the nurse (How long do you think he will live? Do you think I should take my vacation next week to be here when he dies? Should I call the out-of-town relatives to come?). All of these experiences are stressors for the nurse.

The hospice team approach can also be a stressor for the nurse. True team functioning is difficult and time consuming to achieve. There is frequently no clear delineation of functions, and the roles of the team members often overlap. For example, the roles of the nurse and social worker often coincide, and this can create stress for both practitioners.

Organizational Sources of Stress

Most hospices in this country today are still fledgling organizations struggling to establish themselves and to attain financial stability. The financial resources of most hospices are slim, and most pay relatively low salaries and have minimal staffing. Economic concerns are therefore often a cause of stress.

Since hospice is a relatively new concept, there is a certain amount of glamour and excitement for professional persons who associate themselves with a hospice organization and are "in on the ground floor." Because there has been a good deal of media coverage of the hospice concept, the persons involved feel an especially great need to succeed. The high goals engendered by the publicity, the desire not to make public "mistakes" that will reflect badly on the organization, and the relative inexperience of the individual staff members can be great stressors for all persons involved.

The fact that there are still disputes involving the hospice concept and hospice care can also be a source of stress. For example, controversies about the use of large doses of narcotics, reimbursement decisions, living wills, legal definitions of death, euthanasia, and resuscitation policies can all be stressors.

What White has referred to as "organizational incest" can also serve as a source of stress for hospice workers.[7] White describes organizational incest as staff members who meet "most, if not all, of their personal, professional, social and sexual needs inside of the boundaries of the staff group."[8] A small group of individuals who work intensely for the success of a common goal typically develop close bonds. When there is both professional and personal stress, the need for mutual support is intensified. Mutual support and assistance can become a stressor itself, however, when it results in staff members isolating themselves from other personal and professional contacts and supports.

Personal Characteristics

Various personal characteristics of the hospice nurse can be sources of stress. For example, poor self-concept or weak self-esteem, excessive idealism or an underdeveloped value system can all be personal sources of stress when one is faced with a dying patient.

Inadequate professional preparation or experience can be a significant stressor because the hospice nurse is called upon to make many independent professional judgments, frequently without immediate available consultation. A nurse's lack of experience or previous unsuccessful experience with managing personal stress may itself serve as a stressor, because when faced with new and difficult situations the current demands are compounded by unresolved feelings.

Personal problems, the lack of a personal support system, or health problems can also be stressors for the hospice nurse. The nurse's own preexisting feelings of excessive anger, blame, or guilt can surface and function as further stressors when she is faced with the frustrations and tensions of hospice work.

INDICATORS OF STRESS

Like any other phenomenon that human beings experience, stress can manifest itself in many different ways. Both individual nurses and the nursing staff as a whole can demonstrate stress. Physical symptoms can signify stress. Individuals may experience problems with sleeping, weight gain or loss, headaches, nausea, constipation or diarrhea, or feelings of constant fatigue.

There may be behavioral symptoms. For instance, some individuals may become depressed or withdrawn, while others become overinvolved and engage in nearly nonstop activities. Mood swings or extremes in emotions may be evident. Excessive anger and guilt may be manifested in negativism and antagonism toward patients, family members, and other staff members. There may be increased frequency of lateness for appointments, absenteeism, and risk-taking behaviors (e.g., reckless driving, excessive drinking, atypical sexual activities).

Nurses who are experiencing excessive stress often decrease the quality of their patient care. Depersonalization and routinization can occur. Particular patients may be avoided. Deep personal concern is often replaced by intellectualization.

Stress in a staff often manifests itself by a high turnover rate. There is also a tendency to use individual staff members as scapegoats or to project internal problems onto outside sources. Interpersonal difficulties between staff members tend to intensify as workers turn more toward each other for support and place less emphasis on their outside relationships. Marital difficulties, emotional and mental illnesses, and excessive use of alcohol and drugs may also be indicators of stress.

STRATEGIES FOR MANAGING STRESS

Prevention of stress is preferable to treatment. Prevention means developing strategies for minimizing stressors or for increasing employees' defenses against them. The hospice administrator must be sensitive to the potential for stress and make continual efforts to reduce the effects of stressors on herself and her staff. Various strategies for handling stress are useful to different people. Suggestions for reducing stress through personal actions, personnel policies, support services, and opportunities for professional growth follow.

Personal Actions

Psychological Factors. An individual's ability to avoid and respond to stress is, to a great extent, dependent on his or her frame of mind. Making a conscious decision to develop new ways of coping that will reduce stress is an important beginning.

Once this decision is made, varied approaches can be used. For example, setting realistic personal goals is especially important in hospice work. Having realistic goals and expectations is extremely important in avoiding frustration and in getting satisfaction from one's work. Hospice nurses must establish realistic expectations of themselves and keep these in mind when interacting with patients. They must be especially careful not to fall into the trap of promising patients and families more than they can deliver.

It is helpful for hospice nurses to learn to deliberately pace themselves, much as athletes do. An overexpenditure of physical and emotional energy can leave the nurse with no reserves for particularly stressful times.

Distancing is a technique that hospice nurses find especially useful. The nurse can use it to set boundaries between the work and nonwork parts of her life. Developing a habit of mentally closing the door on work-related activities at a certain spot on one's route home at the end of the day can help promote distancing. Using a beeper system, rather than giving out one's home phone number, also allows for more effective control over personal time when one is not on call. Nurses should resist the temptation to give families their home phone numbers.

Developing sensitivity to one's own need for release of tension is another useful technique for reducing stress. Planning routine occasions to talk about one's own experiences and feelings is important. These "decompression" times should occur in the employment setting, should be time limited, and should involve persons who share a mutual trust and respect. Fifteen to thirty minutes of safe "ventilation" with a peer or supervisor can help hospice nurses distance themselves from their work. In some settings a non-health care staff member, such as the office manager or volunteer coordinator, may be a safe, nonjudgmental outlet for decompression.

Life-Style Factors. A healthful life-style includes a balanced variety of components and contributes to the development of sound physical and psychic defenses against stress. A well-balanced nutritional intake helps to keep physiological functioning at its optimum. A sound body is in itself an important defense against stress.

A life-style that includes relaxing activities to balance work efforts is also important. Relaxation can result from many sources, such as gardening, jogging, scrubbing floors, sculpting, reading, playing a musical instrument, playing bridge. Some activities are specifically designed to produce relaxation, such as meditation, biofeedback, or aerobics. Any activity that is interesting, provides for the release of tension, and is satisfying to the individual is relaxing. The nature of the activity is unimportant. The important thing is that the person's life-style includes relaxing activities.

Support Services

Support services for the relief of stress among staff are extremely important in hospice organizations. The roles of the supervisor, hospice team, and consultants in providing support services are briefly discussed here. Chapter 6 includes more information about the role of the administrator and of the hospice nurse.

Supervision. The hospice administrator often functions as a supervisor for hospice staff nurses and as such is responsible for providing support. In her supervisory role, the hospice administrator can attempt to relieve stress for her staff in a variety of ways. During routine reviews of the nursing care plan with staff members, individual nurses can discuss perplexing patient problems and ideas for dealing with them, and the supervisor can make suggestions for improving nursing care and reinforce existing positive efforts. Expressions of appreciation for a nurse's work in a difficult situation or an appropriate decision can be very supportive. Objective and prompt feedback from the supervisor when a situation has been poorly handled is also important.

The supervisor's most important contribution to relieving the staff members' stress is to be available to listen to their day-to-day concerns, frustrations, and successes. Being accessible to staff members, who are relatively isolated from their peers in home settings, is particularly important. The supervisor can also encourage staff members to establish stress-reduction mechanisms in their own lives. She can help them set realistic goals for themselves and help them overcome the tendency to feel guilty when problems can't be solved or situations don't meet ideal standards. Some nurses need encouragement to apply good health habits to their own lives.

The supervisor must be sensitive to the development of stress in staff members as individuals and as a group. Identifying and labeling early symptoms in open discussions is a way of acknowledging that all persons are susceptible to stress; this can be a way of counteracting stress before it becomes severe.

Hospice Team. Hospice team members can help reduce each other's stress through open discussion focused on mutual support. The conferences, which should be held on a routine basis, should provide an opportunity for all team members to recognize each others' different contributions. Group members can provide reinforcement to each other and can work out specific support arrangements as needed (e.g., trading some responsibilities when one person feels especially drained, covering for each other to make it possible for someone to have an extra day off, arranging for two persons to make a home visit to a patient with especially difficult problems).

Consultant. Some hospices hire consultants—psychiatrists, psychologists, psychiatric nurses, or psychiatric social workers—to provide psychological support services for staff members. These professionals can carry on inservice education and staff development programs as well as lead groups using specific stress-reduction techniques. A useful tool for the entire staff is a consultant-directed one-day retreat, held away from the work setting. Held on an annual basis, the retreat can provide the opportunity for staff members to review their own job descriptions, evaluate their own performance, and suggest additions to or deletions from their responsibilities. This procedure can provide an opportunity for all team members to get feedback from other members on their functioning; in addition, the yearly meeting can provide a perspective on the organization's growth.

Personnel Policies

Flexible personnel policies can be an important adjunct to other stress-reduction strategies. For example, providing coverage of job responsibilities so staff members can attend patients' funerals can help promote healthy grieving. Allowing nurses some time off after the death of especially difficult patients provides an opportunity to replenish psychic and physical energies. A policy that requires nurses to use a beeper system or answering service for calls from patients and families protects them from guilt feelings about not giving out their home phone numbers.

Opportunities for Professional Growth

Inadequate preparation to meet job expectations can be a stressor for hospice staff members. Professional growth opportunities can be a means of increasing knowledge, skills, and self-confidence and thus reducing stress.

Because hospice care is a recent phenomenon and most nurses have had most of their nursing experience in inpatient institutions that emphasize curative care, a strong orientation program for new hospice nurses is essential. Routine staff development programs that focus on refining both technical and interpersonal skills used in day-to-day activities are also important. In addition, programs that focus on new therapies, techniques, devices, and ethical issues help keep staff members from feeling professionally isolated. In a survey of 92 hospices, staff members in more than half expressed a need for further training in 26 of 33 issues and skills in the mental health area.[9] The most frequently identified needs were categorized into the following major areas:

> **Patient issues:** Working with the difficult patient, helping patients understand their relationship to their families, and coping with the emotional stress of treatment.
>
> **Family issues:** Special problems of young children, grown children of elderly patients, parents of child patients, and the surviving breadwinner. Helping family members communicate with the dying patient, family reactions to pain and suffering, and emotional support for the family.
>
> **Staff issues:** Prevention of burnout, emotional support for staff, and development of an interdisciplinary health team.
>
> **Interpersonal skills:** Psychological intervention skills, listening and empathetic skills, and information-gathering skills.

The administrator should plan inservice education both to meet the learning needs identified by staff members as well as to stimulate new ideas and approaches.

Facilitating and encouraging attendance at appropriate professional meetings is another mechanism for reducing stress. The hospice organization that provides both time and at least partial funding for staff members to attend hospice-related conferences and workshops is making an investment in the future quality of its services. Patient-care conferences can also be a means of reducing stress and promoting staff growth. Through these interdisciplinary discussions individuals can be supported as well as challenged by questions and new ideas.

The hospice administrator can also reduce stress by encouraging the staff to maintain objectivity about their work through research investigations. Well-designed research studies focused on patient care are needed in all types of clinical nursing. Hospice nurses have some excellent opportunities to collect patient data because they are usually the professional persons with the most continuous contact with the patients. The administrator who facilitates and guides nursing research can make a contribution not only to the personal and professional development of staff members but also to the discipline of nursing.

NOTES

[1] Mary L. S. Vachon, "Motivation and Stress Experienced by Staff Working with the Terminally Ill," *Death Education* 2 (1978): 117-118.

²Hospice of Marin, "Ways to Avoid and/or Deal with Burnout: Staff Selection and Support," San Rafael, Calif., 1981 (mimeographed).

³Balfour M. Mount, "Personnel Selection: Applying the McMurry Principles in Palliative Care," in *The Royal Victoria Hospice Manual on Palliative/Hospice Care*, ed. Ina Ajemian and Balfour M. Mount (Salem, N.H.: Ayer, 1982), 443.

⁴Louis E. LaGrand, "Reducing Burnout in the Hospice and Death Education Movement," *Death Education* 4 (1980): 64-65.

⁵Mount, *op. cit.*, 431.

⁶ELM Services Inc., "Workshop on Hospice Planning, Administration and Financing," Tucson, Ariz., 1979 (mimeographed).

⁷William L. White, "Managing Personal and Organizational Stress in the Care of the Dying," in *Hospice: Education Program for Nurses*, (Washington, D.C.: U.S. Government Printing Office, 1981), 319.

⁸White, *op. cit.*, 319.

⁹Charles A. Garfield, Dale G. Larson, and David Schuldberg, "Mental Health Training and the Hospice Community: A National Survey," *Death Education* 6 (1982): 196-197.

REFERENCES

Beszterczey, Akos. "Staff Stress on a Newly-Developed Palliative Care Service: The Psychiatrist's Role." *Journal of Canadian Psychiatric Association* 22 (1977): 347-353.

Bystrowski, Kathy, and Jennifer Lillard. "Role Strain in Hospice Nursing." *Home Health Care Services Quarterly* 2 (Spring 1981): 51-59.

Donovan, Judy A. "Team Nurse and Social Worker—Avoiding Role Conflict." *American Journal of Hospice Care* 1 (Winter 1984): 21-23.

ELM Services, Inc., "Workshop on Hospice Planning, Administration and Financing." Tucson, Ariz., 1979. (Mimeographed.)

Garfield, Charles A., Dale G. Larson, and David Schuldberg. "Mental Health Training and the Hospice Community: A National Survey." *Death Education* 6 (1982): 189-204.

Hospice of Marin. "Ways to Avoid and/or Deal with Burnout: Staff Selection and Support." San Rafael, Calif., 1981. (Mimeographed.)

LaGrand, Louis E. "Reducing Burnout in the Hospice and the Death Education Movement." *Death Education* 4 (1980): 61-75.

Mount, Balfour M. "Personnel Selection: Applying the McMurry Principles in Palliative/Hospice Care." In *The Royal Victoria Manual on Palliative/Hospice Care*, ed. Ina Ajemian and Balfour Mount. Salem, N.H.: Ayer, 1982.

White, William L. "Managing Personal and Organizational Stress in the Care of the Dying." In *Hospice: Education Program for Nurses*. Washington, D.C.: U.S. Government Printing Office, 1981.

Yancik, Rosemary. "Sources of Work Stress for Hospice Staff." *Journal of Psychosocial Oncology* 2 (Spring 1984): 21-31.

Zerwekh, Joyce V. "Professional Stress and Distress." In *Hospice and Palliative Nursing Care*, ed. Ann G. Blues and Joyce V. Zerwekh. New York: Grune & Stratton, 1984.

Chapter 6

The Role of the Nurse

Barbara M. Petrosino
Marlene H. Weitzel

Nursing care is an essential component of total care for the hospice patient. The hospice administrator assumes the overall responsibility for the quality and quantity of the nursing services. Besides the staffing and support activities described in Chapter 5, the administrator represents and fosters effective nursing in many other ways. This chapter deals with the administrator's responsibility in promoting community relations and in establishing a quality assurance program. Next, it describes in detail the hospice nurse's role in working with primary caregivers, implementing the nursing process, and handling deaths in the home. The final section, on ethical decision making, sets out some of the problems involved in making the everyday decisions that confront hospice administrators and staff members and presents several decision-making models.

THE NURSE AS ADMINISTRATOR

Community Relations

It is helpful if the hospice administrator initiates extensive contacts in the community in the name of the hospice organization with physicians and other health care providers, personnel in doctors' offices, hospitals, social service agencies, and medical supply houses and mortuaries, and representatives of service and charitable groups. Establishing key contacts before there is a need to involve any of the community resources in the hospice services often results in more positive attitudes. The administrator should offer frequent informational programs about the concept of hospice and hospice care if the contacts are to grow into satisfying relationships.

Communications. To a great extent, the reputation and credibility of a hospice is based on the communications that hospice personnel have with persons representing other community resources. Oncologists, radiologists, surgeons and their office staffs, hospital oncology nurses, and discharge planners especially need to experience a feeling of collegiality and cooperation with hospice representatives. Open discussion about shared responsibility for the care of the terminally ill and their families should be encouraged. The hospice's willingness to provide partial services, such as social work, can be a means of promoting cooperation and consultation. For instance, the hospice social worker can provide support services under contract to hospital staff members who experience stress associated with deaths of patients. It must be remembered that referrals and effective care are most likely to arise out of feelings of mutual respect.

Since Medicare-certified hospices must contract for both hospital and respite services, mechanisms must be devised for communication of the patient's hospice care plan and preparation of hospital personnel to care for hospice patients. Maintaining effective communication must be a primary concern, especially when patient care is provided by several different organizations. The combination of institutional and noninstitutional care, 24-hour care by contract services, and respite care services requires a concerted effort by the hospice administrator and nurse to ensure the continuity of care so essential to the patient and his family.

Changing Patterns of Care Delivery. Reimbursement by DRGs is causing many hospitals to discharge patients earlier than ever before and consequently to offer home care services to fill in the gap. This change may result in hospital staff requests for consultations from hospice staffs rather than patient referrals; more hospitals may also initiate hospice services. Communication about the hospice concept will, it is hoped, improve the care of terminally ill persons, both inside and outside of institutions. It is important to include information about symptom control, comfort measures, and care of both patients and families in these consultations.

Quality Assurance

The relative newness and shaky financial position of many hospice programs does not eliminate the need for a thorough quality assurance program. Only through exacting evaluation and appropriate modifications can high-quality care be consistently achieved. The quality assurance program of a hospice should embrace patient care, administration, and staff development. Nursing is included in each of these components.

The hospice administrator is responsible for developing and implementing the quality assurance plan for nursing in coordination with the overall quality assurance plan for the hospice. The plan should include specific standards or criteria, methods of data collection, a time frame for collecting data, methods for assessing the data and drawing conclusions, and methods for implementing the necessary revisions. Guidelines for quality assurance programs are included in the hospice accreditation standards of the Joint Commission on Accreditation of Hospitals.[1] Standards jointly developed by the American Nurses' Association and the Oncology Nursing Society and those prepared by the National Hospice Organization are also useful sources.[2]

THE NURSE AS CAREGIVER

The Family

Because nearly every individual's life is intertwined with that of his family and social support system, hospice care encourages the involvement of the patient's family and friends. Although the family is usually the primary source of emotional support, for some patients it is secondary. Friends, and even animals who are "family," may be more important to the hospice patient than blood relatives. Their involvement is important in meeting the needs of the patient; it also provides an opportunity for their own needs to be addressed. Family members and friends thus often become both providers and recipients of care.

Since hospice care redirects the control of patient care away from the health care system back to the patient and family, the family is considered an equal partner in both the planning and providing of patient care. The family's participation in hospice team conferences is as important as the physical care they provide. This family involvement requires an open, supportive manner by the nurse. The nurse administrator can often foster this approach in nursing staff members by promoting the same type of climate for the staff. When staff nurses are helped to feel professionally secure, are invited to make contributions to the organization's decision making, and their contributions are acknowledged, they are more likely to encourage a family's participation in the patient's care.

In home care, the designation of a specific individual or combination of individuals to serve as primary caregiver has been an admission criterion of many hospice programs. The primary caregiver is responsible for providing care and for coordinating the efforts of others who assist in the care. If a primary caregiver is not available, some hospices are now arranging for 24-hour care through the coordinated efforts of social agencies, church groups, volunteer groups and other health care agencies, rather than refusing home hospice care to the patient.

Assessment. The initial assessment of the patient and family should include all persons who can participate as caretakers, provide respite care, or provide support to the patient and the family. This thorough assessment of family resources will make it easier for the hospice team to organize services for the patient. The assessment process should include a detailed exploration of the physical and psychological status of the primary caregiver. In addition, the caregiver's past coping patterns and support systems should be explored.

About 55 percent of primary caregivers are spouses. Since 75 percent of hospice patients are over age 50, presumably the majority of primary caregivers are also over 50.[3] The nurse must therefore consider the developmental tasks, health status, and physical and emotional limitations of the caregiver and plan accordingly. The strain of 24-hour care on any single individual is significant, and the health of the caregiver must be considered. Respite care should be initiated when appropriate.

In families where the primary caregiver is employed, allowances must be made for work obligations and responsibilities, since the financial drain of an extended illness is often considerable. The hospice team can often help with planning for substitute caregivers.

Learning Needs. The caregiver's learning needs typically include both psychological and psychomotor components. Caregivers must understand the illness and its changing symptoms, be aware of both their own and the patient's fears and concerns, and know what assistance and support are available to them. They must also be aware of their own feelings, which may include resentment, anger, and depression. In addition, they must learn how to perform the technical care the patient needs. The nurse must remember that the caregiver's emotions will influence his learning. For example, fear of hurting the patient may make learning how to give a bed bath a major hurdle. The nurse should use the same teaching principles that she would apply to any other nursing care situation: proceed from the known to the unknown, use meaningful language, provide extensive reinforcement, and correct mistakes immediately.

In a study of 350 hospice patients throughout the country, Petrosino found that 26 percent of the primary caregivers were men.[4] Nurses should be sure that they are not assuming that caregivers will demonstrate traditional "female" behaviors and roles. Both male and female caregivers may be unfamiliar or uncomfortable with physical care and nurturing activities without extensive guidance and direction.

Family Coping. The patient's diagnosis, treatment, and terminal stage care often require changes in a family's structure, pattern of living, and role assignments, both on a long-term basis as well as in day-to-day activities. Therefore flexibility and adaptation are needed, from each member as well as from the family as a unit. All family members should understand the changes that are needed in order for the care plan to be effective. This underscores the need to involve all individuals in the initial assessment and for open communication among all members of the family.

The family should be aware of the variety of emotions that tend to surface at various stages of the patient's illness, which may include anger, guilt, fear, depression, relief, and satisfaction. Family members need to expect and accept these feelings in themselves and in each other. They should also know that some individuals express feelings openly, whereas others withdraw and avoid the patient and other members of the family. These variations in behavior are normal and not unusual.

The family usually needs to strengthen existing defenses and develop new coping strategies. The hospice team's effort is directed toward helping family members adapt. Participating in the patient's care often promotes coping. Whenever possible, the patient's care should include the participation of all family members, including young children and adolescents.

Careful observation of a child's response to the expected death of a family member is important. School and behavior problems, attention-getting behavior, disturbances in eating and sleeping patterns, hostility, and depression may all arise, and these symptoms may indicate a need for increased or decreased involvement in care of the patient. Generally, children who are involved in the care of dying relatives show signs of less traumatic adjustment to the loss.

Community Support. Existing community agencies and groups can provide physical, emotional, and some financial support to the caregiver. Services such as Meals-on-Wheels, homemaker services, and nursing aides for respite care can be important adjuncts to the caregiver's activities. Small grants from foundations, businesses, and church groups may be elicited for special equipment, supplies, or services. Emotional support may be obtained from various groups, such as the family's church, hospice volunteers, and organizations such as Make Today Count, I Can Cope, Cansurmount, and Candlelighters. It has been well documented that emotional support improves coping abilities and contributes to physical and mental health. Gottlieb and MacElveen provide helpful information for assessing the support available to both patients and families.[5]

The Nursing Process in Hospice Care

The hospice administrator does not generally provide extensive direct patient care. However, because of her comprehensive responsibilities, she frequently provides guidance and consultation to hospice staff nurses and the hospice team. The team is responsible for determining the overall plan of care for the patient, but each health care professional is expected to assume responsibility for appropriate aspects of care.

The nursing process provides a logical and realistic approach to the delivery of effective nursing care. The essential components of the nursing process are the same when applied to the terminally ill patient as to any other patient. A brief review of the nursing process and some factors for consideration will be presented here.

Assessment and Nursing Diagnosis. Assessment is the process of determining a nursing diagnosis from the collection and analysis of information about the patient and his family. The nursing diagnosis then provides the basis for planning the nursing care.

The assessment is always guided by the values and priorities of the persons involved. Sometimes different people—the patient, the family, the nurse—have different needs and goals. If this is the case, all those concerned should discuss the differences in order to reach a resolution.

All aspects of the patient and family's situation must be considered—physical, psychosocial, spiritual, and financial. Depending on the patient's condition and other factors, it may be decided to defer certain parts of the assessment (e.g., intrusive aspects of the physical exam).

Often the initial assessment is done jointly by the nurse and social worker, because their concerns often overlap and their combined expertise can give a thorough picture of the status of the patient and family. For instance, the patient's physical pain may be intensified by uncertainty about health care expenses. Both the nurse and the social worker may need to assess this aspect of the situation. A joint initial assessment also introduces the patient and family to the hospice-team concept from the beginning of their care. Since the initial assessment is generally quite extensive and can take several hours, the patient's condition should determine if it can be accomplished in one visit. Sometimes several visits may be needed. When the patient is in pain, this becomes the focus of the first visit, since relief of pain is a priority.

Published asessment tools can be used to direct the interview or as questionnaires to be completed by the patient or caretaker. Assessment instruments modified for the dying patient are included in Zerwekh's work.[6] Melzack has developed an excellent assessment tool for the evaluation of pain.[7] The nurse must remember that any assessment tool, no matter how comprehensive or useful, should be evaluated for necessary alterations to fit the particular situation. The assessment instrument should merely serve as a guide for the person doing the assessment.

The needs of the family members, especially the caretaker, should be assessed individually, as well as the needs of the family as a unit.

Interactions between individual family members and the patient and between the family members are all important.

The nurse needs finely tuned skills in questioning, observing, listening, interrelating, interpreting, and judging. Well-developed interpersonal and physical-exam skills and clinical judgment are absolutely essential. For example, it may not be immediately apparent that the patient is in severe pain: the patient might have adapted to it, or both the patient and the family members are afraid to acknowledge pain because they are frightened of its implications, or they might not want to complain because everyone is trying so hard to help them. The nurse must gradually uncover such problems.

Terminally ill patients have varied nursing care needs. However, researchers have identified frequently occurring problems in these persons. At least four independent studies cite the common occurrence of the following nursing problems in the terminally ill: pain, anorexia, fatigue, nausea, dyspnea, and constipation. In addition, three of these four researchers also identified insomnia and mood depression as frequent problems.[9]

For more than a decade, the National Group for the Classification of Nursing Diagnoses has been working on developing and refining a taxonomy of nursing diagnoses to further consistency, communication, and research in nursing.[10] The commonly occurring nursing problems of hospice patients mentioned above fit readily into the diagnostic categories. The staff of the Hospice of Seattle have altered some of the psychosocial diagnoses of the national group to make them more relevant to the dying patient.[11] By promoting the careful and consistent use of nursing diagnosis, the administrator can lay the groundwork for nursing research in her agency.

Planning. Planning is the process of developing an outline or design for providing nursing care for the patient and family. The nursing care plan, including goals and projected interventions, provides the basis for implementation. The nursing care must be coordinated with the total care plan for the patient, so it must be consistent with the hospice team's plan.

Goals of nursing care should be realistic and measurable, should reflect the nursing diagnosis, and should be consistent with the values and priorities of the patient and family. Because evaluation, a later phase of the nursing process, always focuses on the stated goals of care, it is extremely important that the goals be appropriate to the situation. For example, increasing food or fluid intake or preventing decubitus ulcers may be unrealistic goals for some terminally ill patients.

The goals should also reflect anticipated problems. The nurse can use her knowledge to project probable future problems (e.g., bleeding, confusion, coma). Preparing the patient and family helps to reduce their distress when the patient's condition changes or deteriorates.

Making a decision about the nursing interventions to be used implies that various alternatives have been considered. There is no single nursing measure that will alleviate a given problem for all patients, so the nurse must consider as broad a range of reasonable options as possible. The selected interventions must be related to the stated goals and appropriate in terms of the constraints imposed by the patient's and the caregiver's preferences and available resources of energy, skills, money, and supplies and equipment. Because the caregiver is generally not a professional health care provider, simplicity is often a useful criterion for deciding on the nursing interventions.

Analysis of the symtom or problem from the standpoint of the causative or impinging factors can often suggest interventions that may alleviate the problem. For example, insomnia caused by muscle strain secondary to splinting efforts should be treated differently from insomnia caused by concerns about relationships among family members. Asking the patient or family what has worked or not worked under similar circumstances in the past also often produces helpful information.

The nurse works closely with the physician and performs an essential role in the relief of pain for hospice patients. She frequently identifies discomfort and its causes, suggests and selects relief approaches, and, especially, titrates drugs according to an overall plan.

Many nurses have had most of their professional experience in acute care facilities and have been exposed primarily to acute pain and traditional ways of dealing with it. Those nurses new to hospice work, therefore, often need guidance in overcoming their stereotyped views about pain and its control. They may need to refine their techniques for assessing and teaching about pain, as well as to acquire new knowledge and skills for the effective treatment of chronic pain. Especially important is the ability to discuss the patient and family's possible fears of addiction.

There are many approaches to treating pain, including transcutaneous electric nerve stimulation [TENS], nerve blocks, acupuncture, radiation, chemotherapy, various combinations of drugs, hypnosis, imaging, exercises, therapeutic music and touch, and meditation. Any one of these approaches can be used separately or in combination with others. Depending on the patient's and family's preferences, a decision may have to be made between invasive and noninvasive approaches. The nurse needs to be creative and open to as many possibilities as possible. Close working relationships among the patient, family, and hospice team are essential to careful exploration of alternatives and appropriate implementation.

When drug therapy is used, the following guidelines should be kept in mind:[12]

> Whenever possible, drugs should be selected on the basis of the cause of the pain (e.g., pressure from inflammation, nerve exposure).

Opiate narcotic analgesics (e.g., morphine, Dilaudid) are recommended for moderate to severe pain, whereas milder analgesics (e.g., aspirin, Tylenol) are suggested for less severe pain. A combination of narcotics and aspirin is effective for many patients.

Much larger doses of narcotics than those used for acute pain are typically necessary to relieve chronic pain. The doses must be adjusted according to the route of administration. For example, rectal suppositories containing large doses of narcotics can be prepared by pharmacists.

Oral liquid preparations should be used whenever possible. (Commercially prepared elixir of morphine is widely used.)

Titration of the dosage and timing of the drugs to the patient's symptoms are extremely important. The goal is to relieve the patient's symptoms while maintaining clear mentation.

Drugs should be administered on a regular, never p.r.n., basis to keep the patient comfortable and prevent the recurrence of pain. Families often need reinforcement of the need for this procedure.

Combining drugs can be useful in eliminating side-effects of other therapies or multiple symptoms (e.g., tranquilizers with morphine to relieve the nausea frequently associated with it, tranquilizers with narcotics to potentiate effects and relieve anxiety, stool softeners with narcotics to minimize constipation).

Drug addiction is highly unlikely in terminally ill patients, and drug tolerance and dependence are not major problems.

Implementation. Implementation is the process of providing the nursing care specified in the plan. In hospice care the nurse usually does not perform all direct patient care herself. Rather, the caregiver or home health aide generally carries out the planned interventions. The nurse is responsible for teaching the caregiver and others how to perform the activities.

In teaching the caregiver, the nurse should emphasize that interventions or activities are a means to the end, the achievement of the stated goals. By stressing the goals, the tendency of a nonprofessional to try to do everything "exactly the way the nurse did it" is avoided. Both the caregiver and the patient should clearly understand the goals and essential components of the activity. If they do, then modifying or adjusting the interventions becomes the mere "fine tuning" that is expected in working toward any goal. Flexibility is a key to realistic patient care.

The nurse should help both the caregiver and the patient feel as secure as possible about implementing the plan. Clear explanations of directives, expected results, danger signals, how and what to record, and whom to call with questions or in an emergency are all important pieces of information to include in teaching. By using nontechnical language, encouraging the caregiver to demonstrate technical skills, providing praise and reinforcement, and encouraging questions, the nurse contributes to the building of confidence. Initially the nurse should check with the patient and caregiver through frequent phone calls and visits. The frequency of checking can be reduced as the patient and caregiver become more comfortable with the care plan.

Evaluation. Evaluation is the process of determining the effectiveness of the nursing care that has been provided. The evaluation is the basis for making necessary alterations in the plan. The responses of the patient and family to the nursing interventions provide the data for appraising the achievement, or lack thereof, of the nursing care goals. Asking for input from the patient and caregiver will generally provide much of the necessary information. When goals are being achieved, implementation of the current plan is continued. When goals have not been achieved or have been only partially achieved, different interventions may be considered or the goal itself may be revised. The nursing evaluation is a component of the evaluation of the patient's total care. Therefore, results of the evaluation should be communicated to the hospice team.

Table 6.1 includes samples of nursing problems frequently seen in terminally ill patients, along with corresponding nursing diagnoses, nursing goals, alternate nursing interventions, and evaluations of the goals. The nursing diagnoses are taken from the work of the National Group for the Classification of Nursing Diagnoses.[13] Because of space limitations, Table 6.1 does not include mention of any specific drugs. Many references are available for this information.[14]

Death in the Home

The hospice nurse may be present at the death of a patient or shortly thereafter. Often, when the death is peaceful and anticipated the family will not notify the hospice nurse until the patient has died. At that time the family's status should be evaluated; a home visit may or may not be necessary. In other situations the family will want the nurse to be present as the patient is dying, and she can then observe the reactions of the family members. In either case a predetermined list of persons to be notified and other steps to be followed should guide the family's actions. The family's wish to stay with the deceased, await the arrival of relatives or clergy, or even groom the body should be respected.

Since established procedures on deaths in the home vary according to state and local regulations, a local funeral director is the most reliable source of information on these matters. Funeral directors have established

TABLE 6.1
THE NURSING PROCESS IN HOSPICE CARE: EXAMPLES

Nursing Problem	Nursing Diagnoses[a]	Nursing Goals	Suggested Nursing Interventions	Nursing Goal Evaluations
Fatigue, weakness	Activity intolerance	Patient will increase tolerance of activity to be able to perform own personal hygiene	Plan rest alternating with activity Select activities to conserve energy Passive–active range of motion Supportive equipment (e.g., walker, commode, handrails, shower seat)	Patient brushing own teeth and washing face and hands after six days
Constipation	Bowel elimination, alteration in: constipation	Patient will have regular bowel elimination at least every third day	Prevention efforts whenever possible Consistent elimination pattern Increased fluid and fiber intake Sitting position for defecation Increased activity Stool softeners, laxatives, suppositories Enemas	Patient evacuated hard fecal material with extreme difficulty on Monday, on Thursday softer material evacuated
Dyspnea	Breathing pattern ineffective	Patient will express decreased fear about suffocation	Semi-Fowler position whenever possible Postural drainage Reassurance and teaching Calm environment Oral hygiene Relaxation exercises Someone remaining with the patient	Patient talking more readily and says he doesn't feel so worried about his breathing the last few days

(*Continued next page*)

Table 6.1 Continued

Nursing Problem	Nursing Diagnoses[a]	Nursing Goals	Suggested Nursing Interventions	Nursing Goal Evaluations
Pain, restlessness	Comfort, alteration in	Patient will be comfortable enough to interact daily in a satisfying manner with family members	Hot or cold applications Position changes Massage, acupuncture Imagery Hypnosis Relaxation exercises Therapeutic touch Music Calm environment Psychological, spiritual counseling Someone remaining with the patient	Patient says she's now able to talk with her grandson about the school activities he's involved in when he stops to visit each afternoon
Depression, anxiety	Coping, ineffective: individual	Patient will voluntarily participate in conversations with family members	Psychological, spiritual counseling Occupational therapy Teach normal grief and coping strategies Imagery Provide increased opportunities for decision making Encourage setting of short-term goals Control physical symptoms	Patient initiating short conversations with family members when they visit
Depression, anxiety, disorganization, fatigue (of family)	Coping, ineffective: family	Wife and daughter will express feelings of managing satisfactorily	Psychological, spiritual counseling Teach about normal grief reactions and coping strategies Relaxation techniques Set short-term goals Respite care Diversional activities	Wife and daughter both spending at least 1/2 day per week out of house and say they "feel better about things"

Anorexia	Nutrition, alteration in	Patient will express satisfaction about his nutritional intake	Planning around patient's preferences Small frequent feedings Supplemental feedings Relaxing, pleasant environment Alcoholic drink before meals Frequent oral hygiene Rest before eating Upright position while eating	Patient says food is "tasting better," and he's "not so weak because I'm eating more some days"
Nausea	Nutrition, alteration in	Patient will express relief of nausea	Alternatives as for Anorexia, except for alcohol Imagery Relaxation exercises Hypnosis Treatment of constipation Carbonated beverages	Patient states nausea is less intense than before
Insomnia	Sleep-pattern disturbance	Patient will sleep restfully at least 6 hours per night	Relaxation exercises Conducive environment (e.g., temperature, sounds, lighting) Music Psychological, spiritual counseling Backrubs Warm fluids Comfortable positioning Avoidance of daytime sleeping	Wife says patient is sleeping from about 10 p.m. to 5 a.m. with position changes every 2-3 hours

[a]Sources: M. J. Kim and D. J. Moritz, *Classification of Nursing Diagnoses* (New York: McGraw-Hill), 1982; "National Nursing Diagnosis Group Forms Association," *American Journal of Nursing*, July 1982, p. 1040.

policies and procedures that some will waive for hospice families if arrangements are made in advance. The mortician must be assured that the patient has been under the care of a physician who will sign the death certificate.

Often the necessity for the police or coronor to visit the home can be circumvented through prior arrangements by the hospice administrator. In many instances, the physician's agreement to sign the death certificate will satisfy the legal requirements. In any case, the family should be advised in advance about what formalities will be required when the patient dies.

Previously arranged funeral plans can be carried out promptly, and this is a first step in the healing process for the family. The nurse may help the family contact the mortician. Staff members often wish to attend funerals, and this is to be encouraged. The hospice team can be helped to "close the case" mentally in this way, or by hearing a report on the status of the family. Bereavement follow-up is then initiated.

The hospice administrator should see that the patient's medications, particularly narcotics, are handled properly after death. There are stringent local and accreditation regulations which must be carried out.

ETHICAL DECISION MAKING

An ethical dilemma is a situation requiring a choice between equally undesirable alternatives. Nurses have frequently been described as being "in the middle" because they traditionally have been both legally and morally accountable to many persons and legal entities. Typically, the nurse is accountable to the patient and his family, her employer, the physician, the nursing profession, outside agencies such as licensing and accrediting groups, and contractual and reimbursement entities, as well as to herself. At the least, this often results in conflict, because the values and priorities of the individuals and agencies to whom the nurse is responsible often differ. This multiple accountability can itself be the basis for ethical problems.

Ethical dilemmas for the administrator frequently concern the needs or rights of individuals (patients, family members, or staff members) and the fair distribution of limited resources, including personnel, supplies, time, and expertise. Since none of the hospices in the United States are more than a few years old, most are functioning on a financial shoestring. Because the people involved are generally extremely conscientious and committed, there is a tendency to overextend services, thus stretching financial and personnel resources to their limits. The result is frequent struggles to meet obligations and hard choices about meeting needs.

While the hospice administrator usually does not have total responsibility for resolving ethical dilemmas, she must be able to analyze situations logically and reach a defensible conclusion so that she can contribute to the final resolution. The following incidents are examples of dilemmas that hospices often have to address:

> Making a choice between equally qualified patients, one of whom has reimbursement potential and the other does not, when only one new patient can be accepted.
>
> Meeting the needs of overworked staff members when there are patients and families who desperately need support and assistance.
>
> Responding to a potential patient who badly wants and needs hospice services but has no available primary caregiver.

There are no easy answers for any of these problems, or the multitude of others that must be faced by the administrator. However, attempting to analyze the situation rationally and consider alternatives will help the administrator feel more comfortable with the hard conclusions that have to be reached.

Aroskar[15] has described an approach that nurses have found helpful in dealing with ethical dilemmas. She recommends the following steps: (1) collecting a data base, (2) considering questions arising from decision theories, and (3) considering principles from ethical theories. The results of these steps are then examined within the context of the values of the persons involved and the allowable time frame in order to reach a conclusion.

Some ethical problems also have legal dimensions, which must be considered. Laws or judicial decisions may apply to particular situations. Appropriate legal implications should be considered as necessary, but space here precludes such discussion.

The description of a patient situation follows. The Aroskar approach is then used to analyze the situation as an example of how the hospice nurse administrator could resolve an ethical dilemma. The alternatives included are intended only to be illustrative; other feasible actions exist.

Patient Situation

Mr. D is 39 years old and has terminal leukemia. The family consists of his wife, Mary, the primary caregiver, and two children, Kathy, age 8, and Bobby, age 11. Mr. and Mrs. D were previously very active in the children's school and leisure-time activities, such as the PTA, Scouting, and sports. Both children were previously honor students; Kathy has won swimming medals and Bobby has been on the championship soccer team. Now their grades are dropping, and Kathy has had her first C on her report card. Bobby has announced that he no longer wants to go to soccer practice, and his teacher has sent home several notes about discipline problems in school. Mrs. D is fatigued and worried and is trying to shield Mr. D from the problems with the children. Mr. D senses that both of the children are avoiding him and knows that they are disobeying their mother. The social worker has visited the home three times and reports that she has established good rapport with Mr. and Mrs. D and Kathy but has not had any response from Bobby. She says that the Ds have begged her to continue to see Bobby, and she feels that he will soon open up to her. Since you know that under your present system the family has already exceeded the number of reimbursable social work visits, and the financial status of the organization is extremely tight, a decision has to be made about whether further social work visits should be made.

Data Base. Who is involved in the situation, and how are they involved?

Mr. D: knows he is terminally ill and is concerned about his family.

Mrs. D: primary caregiver, worried about her children and husband.

Kathy: frightened and confused about losing her father and the changes in her home life, has verbalized her feelings and views with the social worker.

Bobby: same fears as Kathy but unable to verbalize his feelings to the social worker.

Social worker: wishes to help each family member adjust to Mr. D's illness and to his expected death.

What is the projected action?

Stopping the counseling visits by the social worker.

What is the context of the projected action?

Both children have had behavior changes as a result of Mr. D's illness. Kathy has responded positively to the social worker's visits, although Bobby has not.

What is the purpose of the projected action?

To conserve the limited financial resources of the hospice.

What other alternatives are available, and what are their consequences?

Continue social worker visits until Bobby has been helped to adjust. The result may be that Bobby will be helped but that the financial resources used for him will deprive someone else of assistance; on the other hand, Bobby may not respond to the counseling and the expense will be wasted.

Discuss the situation with Bobby and determine if he perceives any value from the visits and wishes them to continue. By asking Bobby his opinion the potential value of the service can be determined more readily, or he may perceive asking about continuation of the visits as a form of rejection.

Refer Bobby for private counseling. He may or may not receive the help that he needs in this way. Private counseling for one family member means that the hospice team will not be able to integrate Bobby's reactions into the team efforts. Private counseling will probably result in additional expense for the family. Bobby may feel rejected by the hospice team.

Find nonprofessional emotional support for Bobby (hospice volunteer, coach, teacher, Scout leader, clergyman). Bobby may or may not receive needed help in this way. The social worker may be frustrated that she cannot continue her services, and the hospice team may not be able to integrate Bobby's responses into the team effort. Bobby may feel rejected by the hospice team.

What are the probable consequences of the projected action?

If Bobby has no more social worker visits he may successfully work things out himself, which might result in considerable personal growth. However, this traumatic experience might precipitate further emotional problems as he enters adolescence. His parents will probably become more anxious about Bobby and feel rejected by the hospice team.

Decision Theories. Who should make the decision, and why?

The social worker should decide, since she has knowledge of the situation and the necessary professional background.

The administrator should participate in the decision, because she has responsibility for the financial stability of the hospice.

Bobby may or may not be able to decide, depending on his emotional status.

The parents should decide, since Bobby is a minor and they presumably have his best interests in mind.

> The hospice team should decide, because the team members have a comprehensive view of the situation.

For whom is the decision being made?

> Bobby and Mr. and Mrs. D.

What criteria should be used in deciding who makes the decision?

> **Legal:** parents have the authority and responsibility to make decisions concerning Bobby.
>
> **Psychological:** unresolved conflicts or problems typically cause future emotional difficulties.
>
> **Economic:** financial stability is essential to the continued existence of the organization.
>
> **Social:** a service agency has the responsibility to provide essential services to all patients.

What kind of consent is needed from the client to implement the intended action?

> If Bobby does not consent to discontinuing the visits, he may feel abandoned.
>
> If the visits are continued without at least Bobby's tacit consent, the interactions are unlikely to have positive results.

What, if any, moral principles are supported or negated by the projected action?

> Considering Bobby's opinion could enhance his self-determination; ignoring his view could negate his right to self-determination.
>
> Stopping the visits could negate the principle of beneficence (doing good) for Bobby and his parents.
>
> Stopping the visits could enhance the principle of justice for other patients if someone else can then receive services.

Ethical Theories. The next step in decision making is to consider all the information collected as described above in relation to principles derived from different ethical theories (e.g., utilitarianism, egoism, and formalism). The ethical theory acceptable to the individuals in the situation should prevail.

In *utilitarianism,* the determinant for the making choice is the consequence with greatest good and least harm for the largest number of individuals. For example, in this situation the parents, the social worker, and possibly Bobby would be happy to have the visits continued; harm could occur to unknown, unserved person or family.

In *egoism,* the determinant for making choice is the preference or satisfaction of decision maker. For example, the social worker and parents would prefer to continue the visits because in that way their own needs would be met; depending on the degree of pressure placed on her, the administrator could continue or discontinue the visits to alleviate her own stress.

In *formalism,* the determinant for making the choice is the inherent morality of the action, rather than the consequences of the act. For example, the social worker's visits are inherently good and should be continued because they are directed at increasing the individuality of Bobby and the self-determination of Mr. and Mrs. D.

Values. Various values of the persons involved must also be considered. For example, if the parents, social worker, and nurse administrator value self-determination, an alternative honoring Bobby's preference will probably be chosen. If the nurse administrator values adherence to policies and guidelines more highly, the visits will undoubtedly be discontinued. Other values could also play an important role in the decision.

Time. In this situation the time element is not crucial because the action does not have to be carried out immediately. In other circumstances, such as when a decision to perform life-sustaining action (e.g., cardiopulmonary resuscitation) must be made, time is a very important factor to consider.

Decision. Reflecting on the information collected and on ethical theory, within the framework of values and time, allows one to reach a reasoned decision about continuing the social worker visits. The result probably will not be ideal, nor will it satisfy everyone concerned, but the decision will be based on a thorough examination of all relevant information and alternatives.

This section has attempted to introduce one approach the nurse administrator can use to draw conclusions about ethical dilemmas. No easy solutions exist, but reasoned analysis can help the administrator feel more confident. Besides the guidelines described here, review of the Code of Ethics of the American Nurses' Association and work done by a Presidential Commission on ethical problems are recommended as background for considering ethical dilemmas.[16]

NOTES

[1] Joint Commission on Accreditation of Hospitals, *Hospice Standards Manual* (Chicago: Joint Commission on Accreditation of Hospitals, 1983).

² Oncology Nursing Society and American Nurses' Association Division on Medical-Surgical Practice, *Outcome Standards for Cancer Nursing Practice* (Kansas City, Mo.: American Nurses' Association, 1979); National Hospice Organization, *Standards of a Hospice Care Program* (McLean, Va.: National Hospice Organization, 1981).

³ Barbara M. Petrosino, "Nursing Care Problems of Hospice Patients and Families," paper presented at the International Primary Health Care Conference, London, November 22, 1983.

⁴ Petrosino, *op. cit.*

⁵ B. A. Gottlieb, *Social Networks and Social Support* (Beverly Hills, Calif.: Sage, 1981); Patricia MacElveen, "Assessing Social Networks and Trends in Health and Illness," in *Social Issues and Trends in Nursing: Chautauqua 1977*, ed. Edna S. Popiel (Thorofare, N.J.: Charles B. Slack, 1979).

⁶ Joyce V. Zerwekh, "Assessment and Goals of Care," in *Hospice and Palliative Nursing Care*, eds. Anne G. Blues and Joyce V. Zerwekh (New York: Grune & Stratton, 1984), pp. 52-59.

⁷ Ronald Melzack, "Current Concepts of Pain," in *Hospice: The Living Idea*, eds. Cicely Saunders, Dorothy H. Summers, and Neville Teller (Philadelphia: Saunders, 1981), p. 81.

⁸ Zerwekh, *op. cit.*, p. 51; Ina Ajemian, "General Principles of Symptom Management," in *The Royal Victoria Hospice Manual on Palliative/Hospice Care: A Resource Book*, eds. Ina Ajemian and Balfour M. Mount (Salem, N.H.: Ayer, 1982), pp. 187-198; Marilee Donovan, "Pain and Symptom Management," in *Hospice: Education Program for Nurses*, (Washington, D.C.: U.S. Government Printing Office, 1981), p. 818; Petrosino, *op. cit.*

⁹ Zerwekh, *op. cit.*, p. 51; Ajemian, *op. cit.*, pp. 187-198; Petrosino, *op. cit.*

¹⁰ M. J. Kim and D. J. Moritz, *Classification of Nursing Diagnoses* (New York: McGraw-Hill, 1982).

¹¹ Zerwekh, *op. cit.*, p. 61.

¹² Faye G. Abdellah, Bernice C. Harper, and Janet L. Lunceford, *Report on Hospice Care in the U.S.: Information for Health Professionals and Health Care Providers* (Washington, D.C.: U.S. Department of Health and Human Services, Health Care Financing Administration, 1982), pp. 6-7.

¹³ Kim and Moritz, *op. cit.;* "National Nursing Diagnosis Group Forms Association," *American Journal of Nursing*, July 1982, p. 1040.

¹⁴ Ina Ajemian and Balfour M. Mount, eds., *The Royal Victoria Hospice Care Manual on Palliative/Hospice Care: A Resource Book* (Salem, N.H.: Ayer, 1982); Anne G. Blues and Joyce V. Zerwekh, eds., *Hospice and Palliative Care* (New York: Grune & Stratton, 1984), pp. 117-121, 160-176; John J. Bonica, "Cancer Pain," in *The Royal Victoria Hospice Manual on Palliative/Hospice Care: A Resource Book*, eds. Ina Ajemian and Balfour M. Mount (Salem, N.H.: Ayer, 1982), pp. 113-144; Richard L. Geltman and Roberta Lyder Paige, "Symptom Management in Hospice Care," *American Journal of Nursing*, January 1983, pp. 78-85; Arthur G. Lipman, "Drug Therapy in Cancer Pain," *Cancer Nursing* 3 (February 1980): 39-46; Robert A. Twycross, "Relief of Pain," in *The Management of Terminal Disease*, ed. Cicely Saunders (Chicago: Year Book Medical Publishers, 1978); Robert A. Twycross and Sylvia A. Lack, *Symptom Control in Far Advanced Cancer—Pain Relief* (Baltimore, Md.: Urban and Schwartzenberg, 1983); Robert A. Twycross and Sylvia A. Lack, *Therapeutics in Terminal Cancer* (Baltimore, Md.: Urban and Schwartzenberg, 1984).

[15] Mila A. Aroskar, "Anatomy of an Ethical Dilemma: The Theory and the Practice," *American Journal of Nursing,* April 1980, p. 659.

[16] American Nurses' Association, *ANA Code for Nurses with Interpretive Statements* (Kansas City, Mo.: American Nurses' Association, 1976); President's Commission for the Study of Ethical Problems in Medicine and Biomedical and Behavioral Research, *Summing Up: The Ethical and Legal Programs in Medicine and Biomedical and Behavioral Research* (Washington, D.C.: U.S. Government Printing Office, 1983).

REFERENCES

Abdellah, Faye G., Bernice C. Harper, and Janet L. Lunceford. *Report on Hospice Care in the U.S.: Information for Health Professionals and Health Care Providers.* Washington, D.C.: U.S. Department of Health and Human Services, Health Care Financing Administration, 1982.

Ajemian, Ina. "General Principles of Symptom Management." In *The Royal Victoria Hospice Manual on Palliative/Hospice Care: A Resource Book,* eds. Ina Ajemian and Balfour M. Mount. Salem, N.H.: Ayer, 1982.

Ajemian, Ina, and Balfour M. Mount, eds. *The Royal Victoria Manual on Palliative/Hospice Care: A Resource Book.* Salem, N.H.: Ayer, 1982.

American Nurses' Association. *ANA Code for Nurses with Interpretive Statements.* Kansas City, Mo.: American Nurses' Association, 1976.

Aroskar, Mila A. "Anatomy of an Ethical Dilemma: The Theory and the Practice." *American Journal of Nursing,* April 1980, pp. 658-663.

Baird, Susan B. "Nursing Roles in Continuing Care: Home Care and Hospice." *Seminars in Oncology* 7 (March 1980): 28-38.

Benoliel, Jeanne Quint. "Nurses and the Human Experience of Dying." In *New Meanings of Death,* ed. Herman Fiefel. New York: McGraw-Hill, 1977.

Blues, Anne G., and Joyce V. Zerwekh, eds. *Hospice and Palliative Nursing Care.* New York: Grune & Stratton, 1984.

Bonica, John J. "Cancer Pain." In *The Royal Victoria Hospice Manual on Palliative/Hospice Care: A Resource Book,* eds. Ina Ajemian and Balfour M. Mount. Salem, N.H.: Ayer, 1982.

Burns, Nancy. *Nursing and Cancer.* Philadelphia: Saunders, 1982.

Bohnet, Nancy L. "Quality Assurance as an Ongoing Component of Hospice Care." *Quality Review Bulletin* 8 (May 1982): 7-11.

Cohen, Kenneth. *Hospice: Prescription for Terminal Illness.* Germantown, Md.: Aspen, 1979.

Davis, Anne J., and Mila A. Aroskar. *Ethical Dilemmas and Nursing Practice.* Norwalk, Conn.: Appleton-Century-Crofts, 1983.

Donovan, Marilee. "Pain and Symptom Management." In *Hospice: Education Program for Nurses.* Washington, D.C.: U.S. Government Printing Office, 1981.

_____. "Relaxation with Guided Imagery: A Useful Technique." *Cancer Nursing* 3 (February 1980): 27-32.

Feifel, Herman, ed. *New Meanings of Death.* New York: McGraw-Hill, 1977.

Ferszt, Ginette, and Priscilla D. Houck. "Integration of the Community Health Nurse in a Hospital-Based Hospice Program." *Oncology Nursing Forum* 10 (Summer 1983): 36-39.

Garfield, Charles A. *Psychosocial Care of the Dying Patient.* New York: McGraw-Hill, 1978.

Gottlieb, B. A. *Social Networks and Social Support.* Beverly Hills, Calif.: Sage, 1981.

Geltman, Richard L., and Roberta Lyder Paige. "Symptom Management in Hospice Care." *American Journal of Nursing,* January 1983, pp. 78-85.

Hamilton, Michael P., and Helen F. Reid, eds. *A Hospice Handbook: A New Way to Care for the Dying.* Grand Rapids, Mich.: Eerdmans, 1980.

Joint Commission on Accreditation of Hospitals. *Hospice Standards Manual.* Chicago: Joint Commission on Accreditation of Hospitals, 1983.

Kim, M. J., and D. J. Moritz, eds. *Classification of Nursing Diagnoses.* New York: McGraw-Hill, 1982.

Krieger, Dolores. *Therapeutic Touch.* Englewood Cliffs, N.J.: Prentice-Hall, 1979.

Koff, Theodore H. *Hospice: A Caring Community.* Cambridge, Mass.: Winthrop, 1980.

Lack, Sylvia, and Robert Buckingham. *First American Hospice: Three Years of Home Care.* New Haven, Conn.: The Connecticut Hospice, 1978.

Lipman, Arthur G. "Drug Therapy in Cancer Pain." *Cancer Nursing* 3 (February 1980): 39-46.

McCaffery, Margo. *Nursing Management of the Patient with Pain.* Philadelphia: Lippincott, 1979.

McKegney, F. Patrick, Linda R. Bailey, and Jerome W. Yates. "Prediction and Management of Pain in Patients with Advanced Cancer." *General Hospital Psychiatry* 3 (1981): 95-101.

MacElveen, Patricia. "Assessing Social Networks in Health and Illness." *Social Issues and Trends in Nursing: Chautauqua 1977,* ed. Edna S. Popiel. Thorofare, N.J.: Charles B. Slack, 1979.

Martinsen, Ida. *Home Care for the Dying Child.* New York: Appleton-Century-Crofts, 1976.

Melzack, Ronald. *The Puzzle of Pain.* Harmondsworth, England: Penguin Books, 1973.

———. "The McGill Pain Questionnaire: Major Properties and Scoring Methods." *Pain* 1 (1975): 277-299.

———. "Current Concepts of Pain." In *Hospice: The Living Idea,* eds. Cicely Saunders, Dorothy H. Summers, and Neville Teller. Philadelphia: Saunders, 1981.

Melzack, Ronald, Balfour M. Mount, and John M. Gordon. "The Brompton Mixture versus Morphine Solution Given Orally: Effects on Pain." *Canadian Medical Association Journal* 120 (February 1979): 435-438.

Munley, Anne. *The Hospice Alternative.* New York: Basic Books, 1983.

Murphy, Patricia Partington. "A Hospice Model and Self-Care Theory." *Oncology Nursing Forum* 8 (1981): 19-21.

Oncology Nursing Society and American Nurses' Association Division on Medical-Surgical Nursing Practice. *Outcome Standards for Cancer Nursing Practice.* Kansas City, Mo.: American Nurses' Association, 1979.

Petrosino, Barbara M. "Nursing Care Problems of Hospice Patients and Families." Paper presented at the International Primary Health Care Conference, London, November 1983.

President's Commission for the Study of Ethical Problems in Medicine and Biomedical and Behavioral Research. *Summing Up: Final Report on Studies of the Ethical and Legal Problems in Medicine and Biomedical and Behavioral Research.* Washington, D.C.: U. S. Government Printing Office, 1983.

Saunders, Cicely. *The Management of Terminal Disease.* London: Edward Arnold, 1978.

Saunders, Cicely, Dorothy H. Summers, and Neville Teller. *Hospice: The Living Idea.* Philadelphia: Saunders, 1981.

National Hospice Organization. *Standards of a Hospice Care Program.* McLean, Va.: National Hospice Organization, 1981.

"National Nursing Diagnosis Group Forms Association." *American Journal of Nursing,* July 1982, p. 1040.

Stoddard, Sandol. *The Hospice Movement: A Better Way of Caring for the Dying.* New York: Vantage Books, 1978.

Twycross, Robert A. "Relief of Pain." In *The Management of Terminal Disease,* ed. Cicely Saunders. Chicago: Yearbook Medical Publishers, 1978.

Twycross, Robert A., and Sylvia A. Lack. *Symptom Control in Far Advanced Cancer—Pain Relief.* Baltimore: Urban and Schwartzenberger, 1983.

_____ . *Therapeutics in Terminal Cancer.* Baltimore: Urban and Schwartzenberger, 1984.

Wald, Florence S., Zelda Foster, and Henry J. Wald. "The Hospice Movement as a Health Care Reform." *Nursing Outlook* 28 (March 1980): 173-178.

Wylie, Norma A. "Nursing Care of Terminally Ill Patients in Hospital Settings." *Quality Review Bulletin* 6 (December 1980): 4-8.

Winstead, Daniel K., Robert Dollar, Margaret Gilmore, and Elizabeth Miller. "Hospice Consultation Team—A New Multidisciplinary Model." *General Hospital Psychiatry* 3 (1980): 169-176.

Zerwekh, Joyce V. "Assessment and Goals of Care." In *Hospice and Palliative Nursing Care,* eds. Anne G. Blues and Joyce V. Zerwekh. New York: Grune & Stratton, 1984.

Zimmerman, Jack M., ed. *Hospice: Complete Care for the Terminally Ill.* Baltimore: Urban and Schwartzenberger, 1981.

Chapter 7

Volunteers

Diane S. Pedersen

INTRODUCTION

Some ten years ago, professional and lay volunteers were at the heart of the development of hospice programs in America. Freely and generously contributing their time and expertise, they brought about a new trend in the care of dying persons. Inspired by the model of hospice in England, notably St. Christopher's of London, and troubled by the way so many terminal patients in America were dying, these volunteers organized their resources into pioneering programs of support for the dying and their families. From their informal initial meetings in homes, churches, and schools, there grew a grassroots hospice movement that is fast becoming an accepted part of the health care system.

A volunteer is someone who performs a service of his own free will; a hospice volunteer is someone who contributes freely of his time, so that his very presence represents the gift of himself and gives expression to the philosophy of compassionate care that has come to be known as hospice. Although volunteerism is not unique to hospice, it constitutes the backbone and spirit of this emerging concept of care.[1]

The hospice role, moreover, is a new one for health care volunteers. While in the past volunteers have not been viewed as essential to the organizations in which they served, hospice volunteers often serve as founding members of the hospice board and provide direct care as well. "This voluntary dimension of the hospice model has become the hallmark of the movement."[2]

Significantly, volunteers are included in the National Hospice Organization's definition of hospice:

> A Hospice is a program of palliative and supportive services which provides physical, psychological, social, and spiritual care for dying persons and their families. Services are provided by a medically supervised interdisciplinary team of professionals and volunteers. . . .[3]

Large numbers of well-trained volunteers, who augment the services of the professional staff, are crucial to the existence of hospice programs, because hospice provides more than just good medical and nursing care. Because of their numbers and availability, volunteers can provide a good portion of the care. They provide services in ways that other members of the team are unable to. For example, by writing a letter, reading aloud, or holding a patient's hand and listening, a volunteer can offer comfort that the professional does not always have time for. Through these extraordinary caring acts from a stranger who is there because he chooses to be, the volunteer enables the patient and family to experience the meaning of hospice care.

This chapter, which describes the role of the hospice volunteer, does not attempt to address all aspects of the volunteer program. Rather, it focuses on some of the main issues of interest and concern to the administrator who is responsible for developing and managing a group of volunteers. Its concentration on such topics as program structure, contributions of volunteers to hospice work, and the process of recruiting, screening, and training follow from my personal experience as director of two hospital-based home-care hospices.

ORGANIZATIONAL AND FINANCIAL ISSUES

Conflict of Philosophies

Buckingham and Lupu describe two emerging types of hospices: "independent, heavily volunteer hospices" and "institutionally based hospices . . . having fewer types of volunteers and staff. . . ."[4] The first is a direct extension of the community that it serves and may be successful in providing a wide variety of services because it is a separate and autonomous entity whose mission is simple, clear, and straightforward. The second type, especially the hospital-based hospice, is an expansion of services already provided to sick but not necessarily dying persons. Since its mission to give a different kind of care sets hospice apart from other hospital departments, hospice at times finds itself in philosophical conflict within its parent institution in regard to overall purpose (curative versus palliative care). In addition, the established volunteer group within the hospital may neither have keen interest in the unique dimensions of hospice services nor choose to become involved in it. For the institutionally based hospice, then, the volunteer component should be developed within the hospice organizational framework, separate from the traditional volunteer group.

Funding

Buckingham and Lupu further describe the two types of hospice in regard to financial status. The independent hospice experiences considerable funding problems, while "a major advantage of the institutional affiliation is financial support."[5] Independent community-based hospice organizations must rely on the work of volunteers, memorial donations, and fund raising to finance their programs. Unlike hospitals and home health agencies, they cannot receive reimbursement through third-party payment. For this reason, some establish contractual relationships with health care facilities, but in general they utilize professional volunteers such as nurses for skilled nursing care and lay volunteers for nonskilled personal care.

Hospitals and home health agencies, on the other hand, receive payment for most of their skilled services. The right to payment is granted through a license by the state and certification by Medicare. Even within the Medicare hospice program, not all required services are reimbursable; therefore, volunteers contribute in large measure to the financial well-being of all hospice programs.

Certain costs are associated with starting and operating a volunteer program for any type of hospice. First, a capable director or coordinator of volunteers is essential to ensure consistency of service and to assume responsibility for training. Although some programs begin with a part-time volunteer director, as the program grows in numbers of volunteers and patients a paid employee, preferably full time, is needed for the position. Other costs, such as those of office space and equipment, clerical support, liability insurance, and training, may be expected. In addition, travel expenses, publicity, and miscellaneous expenses for special programs should be considered. For example, on "Daffodil Day" each spring at the St. Agnes Hospital Home Care/Hospice, volunteers deliver bouquets of daffodils to hospice families.

ROLES AND RESPONSIBILITIES

Hospice programs need volunteers to perform a variety of tasks. The St. Agnes Hospital Home Care/Hospice Program, for instance, lists a number of volunteer service opportunities under two main categories as follows:

1. **Program Support Positions**

    a. Organizers of the annual hospice fair, an educational forum and fund-raising event.

    b. Public speakers to present program to community organizations.

c. Clerical work, such as editing, typing, filing, collating, photocopying, data collection, and mass mailings.
   d. Individual or group workers for updating mailing lists.
   e. Hosts and hostesses for meetings, conferences, workshops, and social events.
   f. Coordinators for conferences and social events.
   g. Professional nurses to provide inservice training in personal care.
   h. Drivers for errands and volunteer transport.
   i. Babysitters for children of volunteers.
   j. Leadership positions in coordinating volunteer teams assigned to a specific job description.
   k. Psychodramatists, clowns, or actors utilized in ways unique to their special talents.

2. Direct Patient and Family Positions
   a. "Hospice friend" assigned to a patient or family member as part of the regular care team.
   b. Drivers for escorting and transporting patients and family members to appointments and social outings.
   c. Drivers for errands, such as picking up medicine and supplies, food shopping, laundry, etc.
   d. Assistants for homemaking and home-maintenance tasks.
   e. Mental health professionals to aid the clinical staff in the counseling of patients and families.
   f. Pastoral care professionals to provide spiritual counseling to patients, families, and staff members.
   g. Physicians to provide liaison with the medical community and to promote good public relations.
   h. Professionals and nonprofessionals in areas of music, art, handicrafts, and recreational activities.
   i. Bereavement team members to follow families through bereavement.[6]

A large number of volunteers are needed to give direct patient and family care as "hospice friends." These volunteers help care for the dying person by being good and patient listeners and by providing occasional respite for the family. Volunteers who learn to give bed baths and back rubs, change bed linens, or perform other basic elements of good nursing care make a valuable contribution to hospice work. Physical care of the patient at home when the caregiver is out shopping or just having a well earned rest helps the patient feel less of a burden on his family and reassures the family about the patient's comfort and welfare.

Although it is still unusual, a few hospices are now giving volunteers more responsibility for direct care, thus relieving hospice staff members who, through necessity, are restricted by time schedules. The patient and the hospital benefit from this more flexible personal care.

Home care and inpatient volunteer service differ in the scheduling of hours. Since the goal for an inpatient unit is to cover specific hours of the day, volunteers are asked for regular blocks of time. They are assigned to the same patients each time they report for duty. Should the patient return home, home care volunteers may take over. Although some volunteers work in both inpatient and home care settings, most choose one over the other. Some prefer the regular hours of the inpatient unit to the less predictable hours of home care.

As part of the home care interdisciplinary team, the volunteer is ideally assigned to only one or two patients at a time. The goal is to provide continuous support of the same patient and family. Because of the large number of special requests received almost daily in a busy hospice program, however, a group of volunteers is also needed to be available on demand.

The possibilities for matching patients' needs with volunteers' abilities are unlimited, given a large number of volunteers. Most volunteers are selective about what they will do and when they are available. For example, some prefer not to give physical care but are willing to sit with the patient. Others are willing to provide physical care but are frightened by very sick patients. Some can work during the school year but not during the summer; others may need to rest after an emotionally draining case. For these and many other reasons, a number of volunteers are needed in order to find the right one for a specific request.

The number of active volunteers usually fluctuates. Some serve for years, while others soon leave. Although St. Agnes has approximately 50 volunteers, many more could be used for its average daily census of 30 hospice home care patients. Hospices often need to increase the number of potential volunteers by expanding recruitment into new areas.

RECRUITMENT AND SCREENING

Recruitment of volunteers is directed to the communities in which the patients live or to the hospice's service area. Through announcements at churches, advertisements in newsletters, and word of mouth, the potential volunteer learns about hospice and becomes interested in it. The death of a family member or friend often attracts to hospice work a person who senses that more could have been done. For some the caregiving role is a natural expression of religious belief. For others, the impetus is a desire to be a part of a dedicated team effort. For still others it is a response to a need for challenge that will lead to personal growth and a fuller life. People who come to hospice for all these reasons are talented, caring individuals who can use their education and life experiences to do something meaningful for dying patients and their families.

The Screening Process

Beginning with the written application and first interview, the screening process is a combined effort on the part of the volunteer, who self-selects, and the hospice, which observes.[8] The volunteer is requested to attend all of the training sessions. Although training usually focuses on the role of hospice friend, volunteers are free to choose to do something other than direct patient and family care. Volunteers are respected for their unique interests and abilities and are appreciated for their willingness to explore a commitment to hospice work.

The St. Agnes Hospital Home Care/Hospice Program employs a screening process that includes three steps prior to the training program. First is the initial telephone call between the coordinator and the potential volunteer, during which a preinterview takes place. The volunteer's reasons for wanting to become involved in hospice and prior experiences in helping others are discussed. At this time, the coordinator screens out those who are not truly volunteers or who do not currently fit the criteria for becoming a volunteer. Second, the hospice information packet is sent. This includes a selection of hospice readings, a description of what volunteers do, and an application form. The information in the packet allows the potential volunteer to consider certain aspects of the program before the first interview. Third is the interview, in which these criteria are applied:

1. The volunteer has a high school diploma. For reasons of documentation and accountability, literacy is important.
2. The volunteer has had no significant personal loss during the preceding year, such as the death of a spouse, child, or parent, or a divorce.
3. The volunteer is willing to attend all sessions of the training program.

4. The volunteer is asked to commit a specific amount of time to the program, after training. The hours of service are determined by the volunteer.

A second interview with the hospice chaplain, an experienced volunteer, or another member of the interdisciplinary team is sometimes held as well. Desirable qualities in a volunteer include the following:

1. A mature personality with a positive view of life and a view of death as part of living.
2. A gentle, caring approach to people and respect for differences in life-styles and value systems.
3. An ability to listen and to be trusted with personal information.
4. A desire to help others.

Those who appear to impose their religious beliefs on others, or whose emotional needs might take precedence over those of the patient and family, should not provide direct patient and family care. As Joy Ufema explains, we need to have the courage to say "no" to those who are not right for hospice care and "who are seeking to fill a void in their lives by becoming involved with vulnerable, dying patients. . . ."[9] Many people are still in pain from previous losses of their own yet make good hospice volunteers. It is those with unresolved emotional conflicts or grief, who cannot set aside their own needs for those of the patient, who should be excluded.

The screening process continues through the training period and into the period of the volunteer's first contacts with patients. Volunteers engage in self-discovery as they explore attitudes about death. Recognition of their own feelings and those of others helps them decide whether they are suitable to give hospice care.

During a posttraining interview, the volunteer and the coordinator together summarize and evaluate the training experience. At St. Agnes, the volunteer is asked to make the appointment for the final interview. The volunteer's follow-through with this responsibility is taken as an indication of continuing interest. In case the volunteer fails to call, however, the coordinator initiates the contact.

TRAINING AND EVALUATION

Training Programs

Volunteers must be trained before they can function as a member of the interdisciplinary team. This important fact was recognized early in the hospice movement. The first training programs were based on hospices' own experiences and on the writings of Dr. Elisabeth Kubler-Ross on the subject of death and dying, as well as the work of Dr. Cecily Saunders at St. Joseph's and St. Christopher's. The hospice standards developed by the National Hospice Organization in the late 1970s defined the hospice concept and contributed to the growing body of knowledge that was essential to training. Subsequently, a number of training manuals or outlines were published, including *The Connecticut Hospice, Inc.; Hospice Volunteers: A Guide for Training; The R.V.H. Manual on Palliative/Hospice Care;* and the *Volunteer Manual* of the Boulder County Hospice (see References for complete publishing information).

Although training programs vary among hospices, some elements are almost universally present. The primary goal of all training programs is to prepare volunteers to function as members of the interdisciplinary team using accepted principles of hospice care. Training includes both conceptual learning about what hospice care is and experiential learning about how to give it, typically integrated into a 20- to 30-hour curriculum spread over four to six weeks. Most programs include the following content:

1. History and philosophy of the hospice movement.
2. The natural process of aging and death.
3. Physical, emotional, social, and spiritual needs of the patient and family as a single unit of care.
4. Pain and symptom control.
5. Current ideas about cancer.
6. Listening and communicating skills.
7. The volunteer as a member of the team.
8. Feelings about death and dying.
9. Grief and bereavement.
10. Panel presentation by veteran volunteers.
11. Community resources.
12. Field experience with a team member or volunteer.

Most volunteers already possess the necessary abilities for becoming hospice caregivers. Training adds conceptual knowledge and helps refine the volunteer's caring skills. Many training programs utilize role playing, large-group discussions, and small-group exercises to teach volunteers how to care for patients' emotional and spiritual needs. The coordinator or trainer encourages the volunteers to share their meaningful life events with the group, to discuss their fears about death, and to try out ways of responding to situations they may encounter in hospice work. As the volunteers learn from each other and from experienced role models, a sense of identity as a team member begins to emerge. In addition, the group forms a bond that becomes a present and future means of support.

A Competency-Based Approach

My experience in training hospice volunteers began in 1978, when I was a member of the subcommittee on hospice of the Maryland Catholic Health Care Consortium, which is composed of six acute-care hospitals and four long-term-care facilities within the Archdiocese of Baltimore. Because there was a belief that cooperation among members would be an effective way to foster the development of hospice programs, the subcommittee was charged with providing a forum for hospice care, which included the task of designing a centralized volunteer training program.[10]

Since the role of hospice volunteer was a new one and very little work had been done at that time on training volunteers, a core curriculum was developed using a competency-based approach. Starting with reasonable estimates of what volunteers should be able to do, the authors agreed upon four major volunteer roles, or desired competencies: team member, listener-communicator, facilitator, and healer. Learning objectives, which were developed for each planned training session, helped to demonstrate that the competencies have been attained. These 15 learning objectives form the basis for a self-evaluation tool (Figure 7.1.).[11] The volunteer training guide contains instructions for the coordinator/trainer and small group leaders, session outlines, lists of suggested audiovisual aids, readings, and logbook assignments for the participants.[12]

Completing the manual in 1981 was only the first step to organizing a centralized volunteer training program in which the consortium institutions could participate. Support for the joint project among all of its members made the endeavor a success. Costs were kept to a minimum through the sharing of training sites, educational materials, and films, as well as speakers. Programs are sponsored at two locations, one to the north of Baltimore at Stella Maris Hospice, and one to the south at St. Agnes Hospital Home Care/Hospice.

After completing one of several programs offered throughout the year, participants are channeled back to the sponsoring organization for orientation and placement. Both direct-service and indirect-service volunteers must take the training program, because everyone needs to know the hospice philosophy and principles of care. For this reason, staff members, such as nurses, social workers, physicians, and secretaries, may also register when space is available.

Evaluation Methods

True measures of the effects of hospice volunteer training are hard to attain; however, the following methods of evaluation are suggested for use in hospice programs:

    1. The degree to which learning objectives are achieved: The competency profile in Figure 7.1 lists the learning objects that

Figure 7.1
The Hospice Volunteer: A Competency Profile
by H. Richard McCord

This form invites you to rate yourself by placing an X in the column which most accurately reflects where you are now. Please complete the rating before taking the Hospice Training Program and, once again, immediately after finishing the training. It is not necessary to sign your name. We anticipate that a large percentage of trainees will rate themselves fairly low, prior to the training effort. This is natural enough! We hope to be able to demonstrate growth in the categories that follow, by comparing your initial responses (as a group) with those answers you provide at the end of the last session.

	My skills are:				
A Hospice Volunteer Can:	None	Weak	Fair	Good	Strong
1. Understand and articulate the accepted definition and philosophy of hospice team and hospice unit of care (patient/family).					
2. Identify and evaluate the psychosocial, physiological, and spiritual needs of the hospice unit of care.					
3. Identify the relationships which exist among patient, family, and team in a hospice situation.					
4. Distinguish among the varying competencies and needs of each hospice team member and respond to them at his/her level of responsibility.					
5. Identify his/her personal reasons for becoming a hospice volunteer.					
6. Distinguish between his/her own needs and values and those of the patient/family without imposing any one value system or set of beliefs on them.					

should be attained. Numerical values may be assigned to the ratings so that individuals or groups may be compared.

2. **Evaluation of training sessions by volunteer participants:** Use of evaluation forms and a rating scale helps to determine the effectiveness and completeness of each session. The form should be administered at the end of training. Comments and suggestions for future programs should be included.

3. **Patient and family satisfaction:** While it is very subjective, evaluation by the patient and family is perhaps the most desirable measure of the effectiveness of training. Question-

Figure 7.1 (Continued)

A Hospice Volunteer Can:	My skills are:				
	None	Weak	Fair	Good	Strong
7. Identify the messages which a person is communicating verbally and nonverbally and respond with sensitivity, support, and caring.					
8. Identify relationships within a group and the factors which influence them.					
9. Describe his/her role as a representative of the community in the hospice setting.					
10. Affirm dying as a natural process.					
11. Express the meaning of death from the perspective of different faith traditions, especially his/her own.					
12. Identify the causes and expressions of grief in the dying person and in his/her family.					
13. Assist the patient/family through the natural process of bereavement.					
14. Communicate an adequate understanding of holistic healing which addresses physical, psychological, social, and spiritual needs.					
15. Pray spontaneously or formally as requested by patient or family.					

NOTE: Please be certain this form is turned over to the training coordinator at the first session and again at the end of the last session.

Source: Sandra Fink, ed., *Hospice Volunteer Training Program* (Baltimore: Maryland Catholic Health Care Consortium—Archdiocese of Baltimore, 1981), p. C-1.

naires mailed to families from one to four months after volunteer involvement are one way of determining satisfaction levels. Unsolicited letters also serve as an indication of effectiveness.

4. Posttraining evaluation by team members, primarily the primary nurse, to ensure satisfactory performance of volunteers as team members. Some programs do not award the volunteer's training certificate for one year, or until contact with patients can be evaluated. Those who take the course as a means of working through grief or just to obtain a certificate for their resume and are unable to complete the practicum would not qualify.

COORDINATION OF VOLUNTEERS

The coordination of volunteers must be able to give inspiration, support, and guidance to the volunteer staff. The qualifications for the position at St. Agnes include a bachelor's degree; prior experience as a hospice volunteer is preferred. The person should be dedicated to the hospice concept and committed to providing hospice care. The coordination and supervision of volunteer services is of such importance that one of the standards used to assess hospice programs by the Joint Commission on Accreditation of Hospitals (JCAH) lists the management responsibilities of the person in charge. The following items are included: recruitment; implementing a training program; determining need for volunteer services in accordance with the team care plan; assigning volunteers; instructing the team on proper use of volunteers; informing the community about volunteer services; and providing continuing education on a regular basis.

Certain responsibilities may be delegated to volunteers who are able to take a leadership role. For example, a volunteer may help with assignments, collect records, and complete a monthly statistical summary of activities. Others may assist with the details of meetings, inservice education programs, and memorial services. Even if training is provided in cooperation with other hospices, the coordinator is responsible to the hospice director for the overall operation of volunteer services and is therefore crucial to the success of the hospice program.

Volunteers are a valuable resource and should be respected for their services to dying patients.[14] They are appreciated for their individual skills and willingness to give their time to the hospice. They do not expect tangible rewards for their services, but receiving a patient assignment soon after the end of training and being accepted by the interdisciplinary team reinforces their value as caregivers. Utilizing volunteers for the tasks that they have chosen shows that they are needed. Monthly meetings, inservice education programs, participation in patient care conferences, and social events not only serve to inform and educate volunteers but also provide ongoing support.

NOTES

[1] Elizabeth G. Bunn, "Volunteers as the Backbone," *The American Journal of Hospice Care* 1 (Winter 1984): 34.

[2] Vincent Mor and Linda Laliberte, "Roles Ascribed to Volunteers: An Examination of Different Types of Hospice Organizations," *Evaluation and Health Professions* 6 (December 1983): 454.

[3] National Hospice Organization, *Standards of a Hospice Program of Care,* 6th rev., (McLean, Va.: National Hospice Organization, 1979), p. 2.

[4] Robert W. Buckingham and Dale Lupu, "A Comparative Study of Hospice Services in the United States," *American Journal of Public Health* 72 (May 1982): 461.

[5] *Ibid.*

[6] St. Agnes Hospital Home Care/Hospice Program, *A List of Service Opportunities for Volunteers* (Baltimore: St. Agnes Hospital, 1980).

[7] Jack M. Zimmerman, *Hospice: Complete Care of the Terminally Ill* (Baltimore: Urban and Schwarzenberg, 1981), p. 109.

[8] Paul T. Werner, Phillip S. Chard, Carl Hawkins, and Thomas Marshall, "The Selection and Training of Volunteers for a Rural, Home-Based Hospice Program," *Patient Counseling and Health Education* 3 (4th Quarter 1982): 125.

[9] Joy Ufema, "Personal Concerns of Hospice Movement," *The American Journal of Hospice Care* 1 (Winter 1984): 5.

[10] Jo Ann Holback and Sandra Gaut Fink, "Consortium's Hospice Volunteer Training Boosts Professionalism, Cooperation," *Hospital Progress* 64 (November 1983): 45.

[11] Sandra Fink, ed., *Hospice Volunteer Training Program* (Baltimore: Maryland Catholic Health Care Consortium—Archdiocese of Baltimore, 1985), p. C-1.

[12] *Ibid.*

[13] *Hospice Self-Assessment and Survey Guide* (Chicago: Joint Commission on Accreditation of Hospitals), p. 17.

[14] Charles A. Corr and Donna M. Corr, *Hospice Care: Principles and Practice* (New York: Springer, 1983), p. 211.

REFERENCES

Ajemian, Ina, and Balfour M. Mount. *The Royal Victoria Hospital Manual on Palliative Hospice Care: A Resource Book.* New York: Arno Press, 1980.

Baldwin, Marcella V., et al. *Hospice Volunteers: A Guide for Training.* Piscataway, N.J.: Office of Consumer Health Education, CMDNJ-Rutgers Medical School, and Riverside Hospice, 1980.

Buckingham, Robert W., and Dale Lupu. "A Comparative Study of Hospice Services in the United States." *American Journal of Public Health* 72 (May 1982): 461.

Bunn, Elizabeth G. "Volunteers as the Backbone." *The American Journal of Hospice Care* 1 (Winter 1984): 34.

Corr, Charles A., and Donna M. Corr. *Hospice Care: Principles and Practice.* New York: Springer, 1983.

Cox, M. S. *The Connecticut Hospice, Inc., Volunteer Program.* New Haven: Hospice Institute for Education, Training, and Research, 1979.

Fink, Sandra B., ed. *Hospice Volunteer Training Program.* Baltimore: Maryland Catholic Health Care Consortium, 1982.

Holback, Jo Ann, and Sandra Fink. "Consortium's Hospice Volunteer Training Boosts Professionalism, Cooperation." *Hospital Progress* 64 (November 1983): 45.

Hospice Self-Assessment and Survey Guide. Chicago: Joint Commission on Accreditation of Hospitals, 1983.

Lack, Sylvia A. and Robert W. Buckingham, III. *First American Hospice.* New Haven: Hospice, Inc., 1978.

Mor, Vincent, and Linda Laliberte. "Roles Ascribed to Volunteers: An Examination of Different Types of Hospice Organizations." *Evaluation and Health Professions* 6 (December 1983): 454.

Munley, Anne, I.H.M. *The Hospice Alternative.* New York: Basic Books, 1983.

National Hospice Organization. "Standards of a Hospice Program of Care," 6th rev. McLean, Va.: 1979. (Unpublished paper.)

Riddle, Kathryn W. *Volunteer Manual.* Boulder, Col.: Boulder County Hospice, Inc., 1980.

St. Agnes Hospital Home Care/Hospice Program. "A List of Service Opportunities for Volunteers." Baltimore: St. Agnes Hospital Home Care/Hospice Program, 1980. (Unpublished.)

Ufema, Joy. "Personal Concerns of Hospice Movement." *The American Journal of Hospice Care* 1 (Winter 1984): 5.

Werner, Paul T., Philip S. Chard, Carl Hawkins, and Thomas Marshall. "The Selection and Training of Volunteers for a Rural, Home-Based Hospice Program." *Patient Counselling and Health Education* 3 (4th Quarter 1982): 125.

Zimmerman, Jack M. *Hospice: Complete Care of the Terminally Ill.* Baltimore: Urban and Schwarzenberg, 1981.

Chapter 8

Hospice Bereavement Program: Trends and Issues

Alice S. Demi

The hospice philosophy that the family is the unit of care has naturally led to the development of bereavement services as an integral component of hospice programs. S. Lack, medical director of the first hospice in the United States, identified bereavement follow-up services as one of the nine key hospices elements.[1] The International Work Group on Death, Dying and Bereavement included assumptions and principles of bereavement care in its Standards for Terminal Care.[2] More recently the Joint Commission on Accreditation of Hospitals (JCAH) incorporated bereavement care standards as prerequisites for accreditation of hospices[3] and the Health Care Financing Administration (HCFA) required bereavement services for Medicare certification of hospices.[4] Clearly, the leaders of the hospice movement agree on the importance of bereavement care, and the JCAH and HCFA standards provide further support for inclusion of bereavement services in hospice programs.

PHILOSOPHY OF BEREAVEMENT CARE

Bereavement is known to cause physical, emotional, and social stress and in some instances physical or emotional illness. The increased mortality and morbidity of the bereaved are well documented.[5] Since the bereaved have been identified as an at-risk group, efforts should be made to prevent deleterious sequelae. Hospice services provided during the terminal illness and the bereavement period are assumed to facilitate resolution of grief and thereby promote the physical, emotional, and social well-being of the bereaved family members.

Crisis Theory

The death of a family member is a major life stressor which often precipitates a crisis situation in the bereaved. Although Lindemann in his classic study of grief concluded that normal grief could be resolved in six to eight weeks, subsequent theorists and researchers have concluded that death of a significant other frequently takes two or more years to resolve.[6] Caplan proposed that bereavement is not just one life crisis but rather a series of crises that is more appropriately called a life transition period.[7]

Crisis theory, as formulated by Caplan,[8] is based on three premises: (1) the outcome of the crisis is not predetermined; (2) during the crisis, the individual has a heightened desire for help; and (3) during the crisis, the individual is more susceptible to the influence of others than at other times. A crisis is a turning point that may lead to increased health and maturity, or to increased vulnerability to physical or emotional illness, or to social disorganization. What actually occurs is dependent upon the interplay of strengths and weaknesses within the individual and the supports and stressors outside the individual.

Bereavement Adaptation

The Bereavement Adaptation Model (see Figure 8.1),[9] which synthesizes Caplan's crisis theory and Parkes's Bereavement Theory,[10] depicts the interplay of stresses and resources that lead to the bereavement outcome. The death of a family member is perceived as the stimulus that projects the bereaved into the first crisis period, equivalent to the shock and protest phase as described by Parkes. Crisis period II is equivalent to the disorganization phase, while crisis period III encompasses the reorganization phase. The adaptation level attained during each crisis period is dependent on the balance between personal and situational resources and personal and situational stressors. As long as the resources and stressors are balanced there will be no change in adaptation level, but an increase in stress without a concurrent increase in resources will disturb the equilibrium and result in a lower level of adaptation. Conversely, an increase in resources without a concurrent increase in stressors results in a higher level of adaptation, which is evidenced by improved health or personal growth.

Concurrent Crises

In addition to the crises directly related to the bereavement, the grieving person may experience unrelated concurrent crises, such as loss of a job, gain or loss of another family member, or loss of property. If a

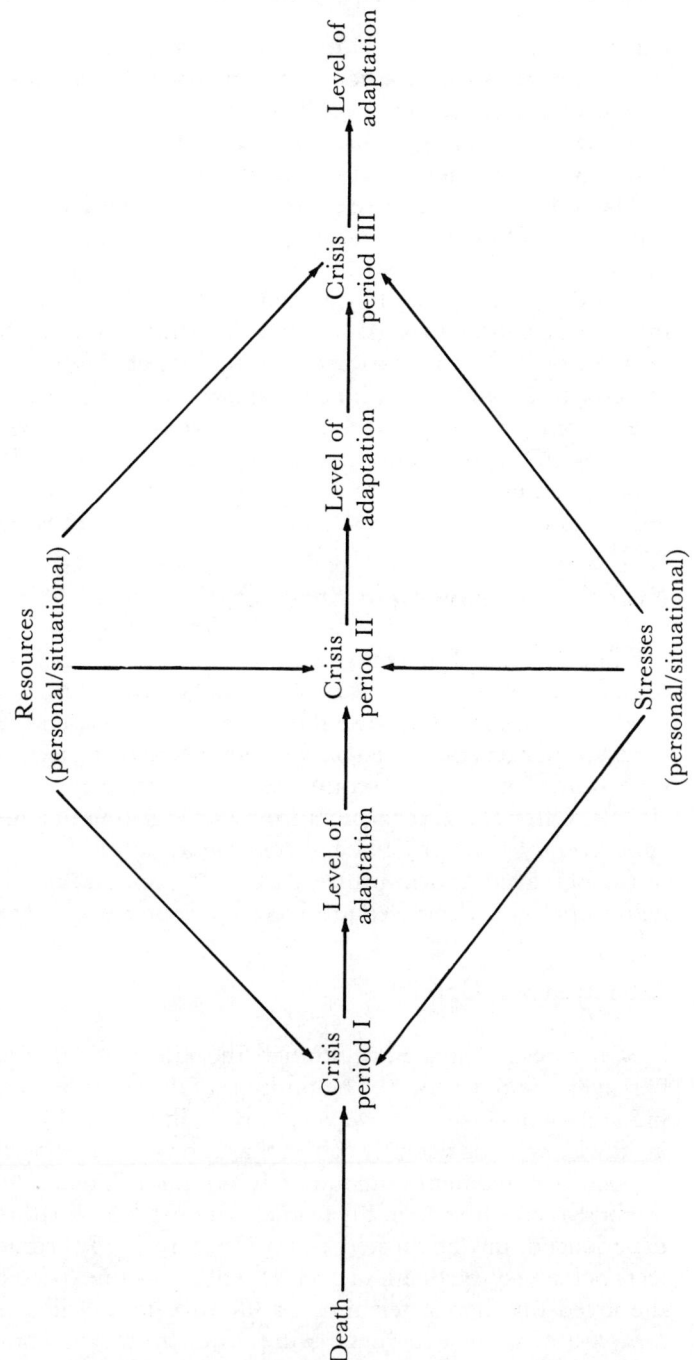

Figure 8.1
Demi/Quayhagen Bereavement Adaptation Model

bereaved person who is barely able to keep his or her resources and stressors in balance experiences a concurrent crisis, this may upset the fragile equilibrium and lead toward unsatisfactory resolution of the bereavement crisis. A similar crisis might have little effect on a bereaved person who has more reserve resources.

The more concurrent crises an individual experiences, the more likely it is that additional external support will be necessary for the bereaved person to maintain a satisfactory adaptation level, whereas the fewer the crises, the more likely it is that the bereaved person will be able to maintain a satisfactory adaptation level without additional external support. In other words, two people might enter the bereavement period with the same amount of inner resources and receive the same amount of environmental support during bereavement but have very different outcomes if one had more stressful concurrent crises. While adaptation to bereavement may continue for many years, the major portion of the adaptation occurs within the first two years for most people.

Need for Bereavement Services

Some bereaved persons with adequate personal and situational resources receive sufficient support from family and friends and therefore need no additional assistance during their bereavement. However, other bereaved persons may need or want additional help, such as that provided by hospice. Still others require assistance from mental health professionals. Often the latter benefit from participation in a hospice program concurrently with professional treatment. In order to meet the needs of the bereaved and to use resources appropriately, it is important to determine which services are most appropriate for each client.

Anticipatory Grief

Many researchers have studied the effect of anticipatory grief on bereavement outcome.[11] The findings of these studies are both conflicting and inconclusive. However, Parkes, in a study of young to middle-aged widows, consistently found that forewarning of death was related to good bereavement outcome.[12] In addition, Volkan found that all of the bereaved subjects in his studies who exhibited pathologic grief had experienced an unexpected death.[13] Interestingly, some of these subjects perceived the death of their loved one as unexpected, even though the loved one had a terminal or life-threatening illness. Clearly, the *perception* of unexpectedness is important to the outcome. Despite the inconclusive research on the value of anticipatory grief, hospice programs are built upon the assumption that services provided to the family members during the terminal illness can prevent or ameliorate unusually intense or deviant grief reactions. Whether the observed beneficial effect of hospice care is facilitation of anticipatory grief or some other therapeutic process is unclear. However, that families that participate in hospice programs have opportunities to engage in anticipatory grief or preparation for the impending grief is undisputed, and hospice care during the terminal illness can facilitate both practical and emotional preparation for the death. Practical preparation includes financial planning, legal preparation, and deciding on funeral arrangements. Emotional preparation takes many forms and may include making amends, saying goodbye, taking a special trip, completing a project, or generally living more fully for the remaining time. While this preparation cannot eliminate the pain and distress of grief, it can make the transition less stressful and is believed to contribute to a healthy bereavement outcome.

Although forewarning and preparation for the death generally contribute to good bereavement outcome, there are many exceptions to the rule. The terminal illness itself may impose special stress, such as uncontrolled pain, disfigurement, and loss of control of body functions. Or the death itself may be unexpectedly distressing, such as a sudden massive external hemorrhage. Or the family members may be emotionally unable to engage in anticipatory grief. Or the family's resources (money, health, and social support) may be depleted by a lengthy terminal illness. Not all hospice families fit the ideal model of consistent, competent nurturing behaviors, open communication, and open expression of emotion. After the death, the bereaved may experience distressing memories of pain, disfigurement, and mental deterioration of the deceased, or they may be plagued by self-doubt and guilt about their adequacy as caregivers. The bereaved family members often feel simultaneous relief, resentment, guilt, and anger.

For many families, hospice services before the death pave the way for successful resolution of grief. For these families, hospice bereavement services are often welcome but are less crucial to outcome. For those families who are less well prepared for the death, bereavement services are more essential to a healthy outcome. The latter families present both the greatest challenges and the greatest reward for the hospice bereavement team.

Goals of Bereavement Programs

How can we know if an individual is making progress toward resolution of grief? The overall goal of any bereavement program is to help the individual or the family unit to move toward resolution of their grief. Worden and Lindstrom each identified four subgoals.[14] Worden stated these goals as (1) to increase the reality of the loss; (2) to help the counselee with both expressed and latent affect; (3) to help the counselee overcome various impediments to readjustment after the loss; and (4) to encourage the counselee to make a healthy emotional withdrawal from the deceased and to feel comfortable reinvesting that emotion in another relationship. Lindstrom expressed the bereaved person's goals somewhat differently: (1) to feel the hurt; (2) to face reality; (3) to achieve a positive memory of the deceased; and (4) to gain a sense of meaning.

Demi, in her description of a program consisting of time-limited semistructured support groups, identified the following 12 goals for bereaved support group members: (1) decrease emotional pain; (2) recognize, express, and accept feelings; (3) increase understanding of the grief process; (4) recognize the normal manifestations of grief; (5) develop healthy coping behaviors; (6) accept the reality and irreversibility of death; (7) develop a support system both within the group and outside of the group; (8) develop a realistic memory of the deceased; (9) promote personal growth; (10) reinvest oneself in life; (11) recognize one's own strengths and weaknesses and seek additional support or therapy as needed; and (12) reestablish a spiritual belief system.[15]

Hospice programs should identify both general goals and specific objectives for their bereavement services. General goals provide direction for the program but are not measurable, whereas specific objectives are more circumscribed and are measurable. Measurement of outcome is necessary in order to assess client progress and evaluate the effectiveness of bereavement services.

Assessing Client Progress

Many instruments are available to measure general emotional distress or specific types of emotional distress such as anxiety or depression. However, there are few instruments to measure specifically the bereavement process or bereavement outcome. Two widely used measures of general emotional distress are the Goldberg General Health Questionnaire and the Hopkins Symptom Checklist.[16] Four nurse-researchers, Demi,[17] Murphy,[18] Rogers,[19] and Vachon,[20] have used these instruments to measure bereavement outcomes. Since depression is one of the major manifestations of bereavement, instruments such as the Beck Depression Inventory,[21] the Hamilton Depression Scale,[22] and the Zung Depression Inventory[23] have been used to assess specific symptom distress.

Several instruments purport to measure the grief process: the Grief Experience Inventory,[24] the Texas Inventory of Grief,[25] and the Present Feelings about Loss.[26] However, only one of these, the Grief Experience Inventory, has been evaluated for reliability and validity. Another instrument, the Bereavement Experience Questionnaire (BEQ),[27] has also been evaluated for reliability and validity. The BEQ contains eight subscales, Guilt, Anger, Yearning, Depersonalization, Stigma, Morbid

Fears, Meaninglessness, and Isolation, Hospice bereavement programs could benefit from use of one of these standardized instruments to assess clients' progress.

Aitken Analogue Mood Scales[28] are another way of assessing client progress. Each scale consists of a line 100 mm long marked at either end with one of two opposite mood states, most sad and most happy (see Figure 8.2). Clients are instructed to mark on the line their perceived mood state right now. Changes in mood state can be easily evaluated by the bereavement team member and discussed with the client if indicated.

Evaluating Bereavement Services

In addition to assessing the client's progress, the hospice program should evaluate the effectiveness of the bereavement services provided. Evaluation should include both process and outcome. Process evaluation should include determination of who receives services, what kind of services are provided, who provides services, how frequently the services are provided, how many referrals are made, and how many referrals the clients complete. The team should attempt to identify any group that is consistently underserved, such as men or the aged. Client outcomes can be assessed by means of the instruments discussed in the previous section. Client satisfaction can also be assessed by means of questionnaires developed by the team. Perceived effectiveness can be assessed through questionnaires completed by bereavement team members. Attention should be given to staff stress and burnout, which can be measured indirectly through staff and volunteer longevity in the program. Multiple methods of evaluation should be employed to gain a picture of both the strengths of the bereavement program and the areas where improvement is needed.

TYPES OF SERVICES

Hospices provide a variety of bereavement services. Some bereavement programs are quite comprehensive, while others are limited in scope. Some provide all services themselves, while others rely on other organizations in the community to supplement their services. There is no one "right program"; each program should be developed to meet the needs of the specific community. What works well in one community may fail in another. This need to adapt services to the sociocultural and environmental characteristics of the community cannot be overemphasized. What works in affluent Marin County probably won't work in the ghettos of Atlanta or the barrios of San Antonio. Even within communities with similar ethnic and economic characteristics, variables such

Figure 8.2
Aitken Analogue Scales

MOOD RIGHT NOW

|⎣ ⎦|

MOST   MOST
SAD   HAPPY

NAME _____

DATE _____

OVERALL LIFE SITUATION

|⎣ ⎦|

POOR   EXCELLENT

NAME _____

DATE _____

as weather patterns, geographic accessibility to services, and availability of other support systems will result in differing levels of success for the same type of service.

Preparation for Bereavement

All hospice programs provide emotional support to the family members during the terminal illness. Efforts are directed toward helping the family members face the reality of the impending death and prepare emotionally and practically for a future without the loved one. Sometimes this preparation is provided by the same hospice team that provides care to the terminally ill person; sometimes a separate bereavement team is introduced early in the terminal illness and continues to work with the family throughout the bereavement period. Much can be done at this time to facilitate later resolution of grief.

Funeral Visits

Most hospices encourage hospice care providers to attend funeral and memorial services held for their deceased clients. Participation in funeral rituals has a twofold benefit. First, the surviving family members usually perceive this as thoughtful, caring behavior and are comforted and supported by the presence of the hospice team member. Second, attendance at the funeral provides a healthy way for the hospice team member to gain closure on a meaningful relationship and to facilitate resolution of their own grief.

Home Visits and Telephone Follow-Up

Usually a home visit or a telephone follow-up call is made during the week after the death. After the funeral is over and family and friends return to their usual routines, the bereaved person may feel grief more acutely and may particularly benefit from talking to a bereavement team member. At this time, the bereavement team member should assess the survivor's level of distress. A formal assessment tool is useful, so that all important areas are evaluated: sleep, appetite and activity patterns, degree of emotional distress (yearning, sadness, guilt, anger), cognitive functioning (confusion, forgetfulness), and actual and perceived availability of support.

Home visits or telephone calls are continued at specific scheduled times and at special dates (birthdays, anniversaries) throughout the first year of bereavement. Some programs do not continue to follow clients if they refuse the first contact or if they remarry. In either case, it is likely that bereavement services are still needed and efforts should be made to continue to provide them.

Educational Programs

Educational programs held on a regular basis (usually monthly) provide a nonthreatening way for survivors to receive both information and support. These programs are often structured so that there is a didactic presentation followed by small group discussion. Survivors who are reluctant to seek "therapy" are often willing to participate in this type of program and may greatly benefit from the didactic presentation and the contacts with the hospice team members and other bereaved persons.

Memorial Services

Some hospital bereavement programs conduct monthly or semiannual memorial services to honor all those who have died in the period since the last memorial service. Hospice team members are encouraged to attend these services with the bereaved family members.

Social Groups

Both formal and informal social groups can meet specific needs of the bereaved. Hospice auxiliary groups or hospice fund-raising projects are often spearheaded by bereaved persons who have benefited from hospice care. Helping others by contributing to hospice helps the bereaved person work through grief. Sometimes hospice reunions, Christmas parties, or other social events are specifically planned to meet the needs of the bereaved, while at other times these are fringe benefits of activities designed for other purposes. In cities where there are social organizations designed specifically for the bereaved, it may be more beneficial and a better use of resources to refer clients to these organizations for social support and focus hospice bereavement services on emotional support, education, and referral.

Self-Help and Support Groups

Many hospices provide support groups for the bereaved. These groups generally take one of two forms: either unstructured ongoing groups open to any bereaved person who wishes to attend the session or semistructured, time-limited, closed groups open only to those who have made a commitment to attend a series of sessions. In both cases, the group is led by one or more experienced group leaders, who are usually licensed mental health professionals or clergy.

Many self-help groups are available throughout the country, such as The Compassionate Friends for bereaved parents, or various widow-to-widow programs such as that sponsored by the Retired Senior Volunteers Program. Hospices usually do not provide self-help programs directly, but they do refer clients to these programs when needed.

Comprehensive Bereavement Services

Large hospice programs with adequate resources may be able to provide a wide range of bereavement services; however, small programs and those with limited resources often must limit the scope of their service. It may be cost effective for them to provide an intensive program to a small number of high-risk clients rather than to provide limited services to a large number of clients. Each hospice must determine what is already available in the community and complement these services rather than duplicate them.

THE BEREAVEMENT TEAM

Hospice bereavement services are provided primarily by volunteers, both professional and nonprofessional. Supervision and direction of the program is generally provided by a health professional who has special expertise in counseling and special knowledge and experience related to bereavement. The bereavement team leader may be a mental health nurse, a social worker, a psychologist, a psychiatrist, or a member of the clergy. Some programs use nonprofessionals in this role; however, most programs find that direction should be provided by a qualified professional.

Nurses who have provided care to the patient and family during the terminal illness may wish to follow the family during the bereavement period. Some families benefit greatly from this continuity, while others wish to avoid people who were intimately connected with the terminal illness period. Families in the latter group may prefer to begin a relationship with a new team member.

Graduate students from various disciplines (e.g., nursing, psychology, social work) often are productive, competent bereavement team members. Families benefit from their services, while the students in turn obtain unique learning experiences. A well-qualified supervisor must be available to guide and support students throughout their clinical experience.

Consultation from a psychiatrist, psychologist, or nurse therapist should be available for the bereavement team to help them work most effectively in complicated situations and determine which clients need referral for more intensive therapy. The consultant may also function as a group facilitator for bereavement team meetings. Usually the consultant is removed from direct involvement with the clients and is therefore able to function as a more objective observer and listener than the bereavement team leader.

Adequate training of staff and volunteers is essential for the success of the program. Most hospices require that bereavement team volunteers complete the general hospice training program before enrolling in the bereavement training program. The training program should include theoretical material on bereavement, group discussion, exercises to promote self-understanding, and role-playing experiences. Training programs range from 10 to 40 hours in length; usually one-half of the time is devoted to didactic material and one-half to individual and group experiences.

Model Training Curriculum

Following is a proposed model curriculum for bereavement team members.

Understanding oneself

Bereavement experience exercises (individual)
Discussion of bereavement experiences (group)

The grief process

Stages of grief
Tasks of grief
Manifestations of grief

Variables that influence bereavement outcome

Individual
Social
Cultural
Environmental
Economic

Helping strategies

Communication
    Verbal and nonverbal
    Empathy
    Respect
    Authenticity
Education
    Grief process
    Grief manifestations

Problem-solving techniques
Mobilizing resources
Coping behaviors

Community resources for the bereaved

Self-help groups
Financial, legal, social, and educational resources
Psychological

Volunteer's roles

Befriender
Counselor
Advocate
Educator
Liaison with hospice team

Evaluation

Assessing clients' progress
Assessing self-effectiveness

Continuing education programs and bereavement team meetings provide additional opportunities for team members to increase their knowledge and skills.

STANDARDS FOR BEREAVEMENT SERVICES

The *Hospice Standards Manual* and the *Hospice Self-Assessment and Survey Guide* were developed through funding by the Kellogg Foundation.[29] Representatives from key professional groups (including ANA, NLN, and NHO) served on the JCAH Hospice Advisory Committee and monitored the development of the standards. Feedback on the standards was solicited through regional conferences, mailed questionnaires, and pilot testing. The accreditation program was officially implemented in January 1984. Several sections of the standards address general principles of hospice care and are therefore relevant to bereavement care, such as the chapters titled "Patient/Family as Unit of Care," "Continuity of Care," and "Medical Records." However, the most relevant chapter is "Interdisciplinary Team Services," which has one standard and several criteria specific to bereavement care.

The JCAH standard and survey criteria specifically related to bereavement services are as follows:

Standard IX: Bereavement services are available as needed to survivors for an appropriate period after the death of a patient.

A. The bereavement services that are maintained to meet the needs of the survivors include, but need not be limited to, the following: (1) regular survivor contact, as needed, following death; (2) an interchange of information between the interdisciplinary team members who provided care before the death of the patient and the individuals who provide bereavement services to the survivors; and (3) a process for the assessment of possible pathological grief reactions that indicate the need for prolonged intervention.

B. Hospice bereavement services are provided by hospice program employees, individuals who provide bereavement services under arrangement with the hospice program, an agency that provides bereavement services under arrangement with the hospice program, trained and qualified volunteers, or interdisciplinary team members who provide direct patient care and have had appropriate bereavement training.

C. The hospice program director designates an individual to supervise bereavement services.

D. Bereavement services are supervised by an individual who has: (1) education and experience appropriate to the care of bereaved individuals; and (2) a demonstrated ability in family and/or individual counseling.

E. Hospice program volunteers or other interdisciplinary team members who provide bereavement services receive appropriate bereavement training. The training program is described in writing.

F. The number, qualifications, and current competence of individuals providing bereavement services relate directly to the skills necessary to provide the level bereavement care required by the survivors receiving hospice services.

G. There are written policies and procedures for bereavement services. Written policies and procedures address: (1) the scope of bereavement services; (2) the manner in which bereavement services are provided; and (3) documentation of bereavement services. These written policies and procedures are reviewed at least annually and revised, as necessary, in accordance with hospice program policy.

H. The provision of bereavement services is based on an assessment of the needs of the survivors and bereavement services are documented and this documentation is representative of current standards of bereavement practice; is goal-directed, reflecting follow-up based on a plan for intervention as agreed upon with the survivors; and submitted in a timely manner, in accordance with hospice program policy.[30]

As part of the JCAH accreditation process, the hospice staff completes a self-assessment of the program before a visit by the JCAH survey team. JCAH recommends that the section of the self-assessment on bereavement services be completed by the bereavement services supervisor. When the JCAH site visit is made, documentation is requested to demonstrate the achievement of the criteria. Direct observation of home visits, team meetings, and other staff activities are essential aspects of the site visit. In addition, documentation of bereavement services is assessed through analysis of written materials, including: (1) policies and procedures relating to bereavement services; (2) job description and required qualifications of bereavement services supervisor; (3) job descriptions and required qualifications of individuals who provide bereavement services; (4) medical records; and (5) the outline of the bereavement training program for volunteers and interdisciplinary team members, if applicable.[31]

The JCAH criteria are stated in general terms, and therefore hospices have flexibility to determine the process by which they will meet the criteria, thus allowing for creativity and flexibility in program planning and implementation. A potential disadvantage to the general nature of the criteria is that subjectivity in interpreting achievement of the criteria may occur. JCAH places great importance on the ongoing development and revision of standards and solicits input for standards from national and specialty organizations and experts in the field. Whether or not hospices seek JCAH accreditation, the development of the JCAH standards and self-assessment guide have the potential to improve the quality of hospice bereavement services.

CONCERNS AND ISSUES

A major concern in hospices is the lack of monetary support for bereavement programs. Although a hospice must provide bereavement services in order to receive JCAH accreditation and HCFA reimbursement, bereavement services are not generally reimbursable. Some hospices have received special grants to support their programs. Inadequate funding places a severe strain on program directors. When funding is short, it is often bereavement services that are curtailed first.

A rapidly increasing caseload is a second concern. For each patient who dies, there is at least one bereaved survivor to be followed, and often there are several. If team members provide both terminal illness care and bereavement care, they may soon be so overloaded with clients that they are unable to provide adequate services to all. Usually, terminal illness care is perceived as most urgent and therefore is given highest priority; thus the bereaved survivors may be neglected. Separation of the bereavement team from the terminal illness team may ameliorate this problem but create another, that of lack of continuity of care. Each program must weigh the advantages and disadvantages of a single team or dual teams.

The appropriate use of bereaved persons as bereavement team members is an issue. Some hospices require that team members be at least one year post-bereavement in order to serve on the bereavement team. More recently bereaved persons may be useful in self-help roles: while helping others they are also helping themselves. However, there is the risk that bereaved persons may be too needy and too vulnerable themselves to function adequately. Hospice programs must carefully evaluate the pros and cons of permitting bereaved volunteers to serve on the bereavement team.

Continuity of care is another issue. How can continuity be ensured when two teams are utilized? Methods of communication must be developed so that the terminal illness team members can share information with the bereavement team members. Adequate record keeping is essential, and these records must be readily available for team members' use.

Who should receive services? All bereaved survivors or those at greatest risk? Money and manpower are not so abundant that all people can receive intensive bereavement services. Hospices must carefully consider what is the most cost-effective way of delivering bereavement services.

The last area of concern is evaluation and research. Very little research has been conducted to date on hospice bereavement programs. Studies should be conducted to evaluate the effectiveness of specific interventions. Clients' short-term and long-term outcomes should be assessed, and more work should be done to identify predictors of outcomes. Clinical observation seems to show that bereavement programs are indeed useful, but hard data are needed to support requests for funding and to guide practice with the bereaved.

SUMMARY

Bereavement services are an integral component of hospice care. Many hospices provide a wide variety of bereavement services designed to ease the client's course through the grief process and to promote healthy outcomes. While clinical observations tend to support the effectiveness of these services, program evaluation and client-centered research are necessary. The development of standards for bereavement care is an important step in ensuring that programs provide a satisfactory level of care. Hospice bereavement services have the potential to improve the mental health and well-being of the bereaved and thereby become an important primary prevention service. Bereavement care exemplifies the full circle of hospice care, moving from care of the dying to care of the living.

NOTES

[1] S. Lack, *Philosophy and Organization of a Hospice Program* (New Haven, Conn.: Hospice New Haven, 1978).

[2] International Work Group on Death, Dying and Bereavement, "Assumptions and Principles Underlying Standards for Terminal Care," *American Journal of Nursing* (February 1979): 296-297.

[3] Joint Commission on Accreditation of Hospitals (JCAH), *Hospice Self-Assessment and Survey Guide* (Chicago, Ill.: Joint Commission on Accreditation of Hospitals, 1983); *Hospice Standards Manual* (Chicago, Ill.: Joint Commission on Accreditation of Hospitals, 1983).

[4] Health Care Financing Administration, *Federal Register*, August 22, 1983.

[5] P. Clayton, "The Clinical Morbidity of the First Year of Bereavement: A Review," *Comprehensive Psychiatry* 14 (1973): 151-157; G. Epstein, L. Weitz, H. Roback, and E. McKee, "Research on Bereavement: A Selective and Critical Review," *Comprehensive Psychiatry* 16 (1975): 537-546; A. Kraus and A. Lilienfeld, "Some Epidemiologic Aspects of the High Mortality Rate in the Young Widowed Group," *Journal of Chronic Disease* (1959): 207-217; A. Maddison and A. Viola, "The Health of Widows in the Year Following Bereavement," *Journal of Psychosomatic Research* 12 (1968): 297-306; C. M. Parkes, "The Effects of Bereavement on Physical and Mental Health: A Study of the Case Records of Widows," *British Medical Journal* 2 (1964): 274-280.

[6] E. Lindemann, "Symptomatology and Management of Acute Grief," *American Journal of Psychiatry* 101 (1944): 141-148.

[7] G. Caplan, *Principles of Preventive Psychiatry* (New York: Basic Books, 1964).

[8] G. Caplan, "Foreword," in *The First Year of Bereavement,* in I. Glick, R. Weiss and C. M. Parkes (eds.) (New York: John Wiley & Sons, 1974).

[9] M. Quayhagen and A. Demi, "Bereavement and Aging, Ethnic and Sex Differences: A Pilot Study," 1979 (unpublished paper).

[10] C. M. Parkes, *Bereavement: Studies of Grief in Adult Life* (New York: National League for Nursing, 1972).

[11] R. Fulton and D. Gottesman, "Anticipatory Grief: A Psychosocial Concept Reconsidered," *British Journal of Psychiatry* 137 (1980): 45-54; B. Schoenberg, A. Carr, A. Kutscher, D. Peretz, and I. Goldberg (eds.), *Anticipatory Grief* (New York: Columbia University Press, 1974); I. Gerber, R. Rusalem, N. Hannon, D. Batten, and A. Arkin, "Anticipatory Grief and Aged Widows and Widowers," *Journal of Gerontology* 30 (1974): 225-229; J. F. Ball, "Widow's Grief: Impact of Age and Mode of Death," *Omega: Journal of Death and Dying* 8 (1977): 307-333.

[12] I. Glick, R. Weiss, and C. M. Parkes, *The First Year of Bereavement* (New York: John Wiley & Sons, 1974); C. M. Parkes, "Determinants of Outcome Following Bereavement," *Omega: Journal of Death and Dying* 6 (1975): 302-323; C. M. Parkes and R. Weiss, *Recovery from Bereavement* (New York: Basic Books, 1983).

[13] V. Volkan, "The Linking Objects of Pathological Mourners," *Archives of General Psychiatry* 27 (1972): 215-221; V. Volkan, "Typical Findings in Pathologic Grief," *Psychiatric Quarterly* 44 (1970): 231-250.

[14] J. Worden, *Grief Counseling and Grief Therapy* (New York: Springer, 1982); B. Lindstrom, "Operating a Hospice Bereavement Program," in C. Corr and D. Corr (eds.), *Hospice Care: Principles and Practices* (New York: Springer, 1983).

[15] A. Demi, *Bereavement Support Groups: Leadership Manual* (Denver, Colo.: Grief Education Institute, 1981).

[16] D. Goldberg, *The Detection of Psychiatric Illness by Questionnaire* (London: Oxford University Press, 1972); L. Derogatis, R. Lipman, K. Rickels, E. Uhlenhuth, and L. Covi, "The Hopkins Symptom Checklist (HSCL): A Self-Report Symptom Inventory," *Behavioral Science* 19 (1974): 1-15.

[17] A. Demi, "Adjustment to Widowhood After a Sudden Death: Suicide and Non-Suicide Survivors Compared," in M. Batey (ed.), *Communicating Nursing Research* (Boulder, Colo.: WICHE, 1978); A. Demi, "Mental Health of Widows After a Sudden Death: Suicide and Non-Suicide Survivors Compared," *Proceedings of the Tenth International Congress for Suicide Prevention and Crisis Intervention*, Ottawa, Canada, 1979; A. Demi, "Social Adjustment of Widows After a Sudden Death: Suicide and Non-Suicide Survivors Compared," *Death Education* (in press).

[18] S. Murphy, "After Mount St. Helens: Disaster Stress Research," *Journal of Psychosocial Nursing and Mental Health Services* 22 (July 1984): 8-18.

[19] J. Rogers, A. Sheldon, C. Barwick, K. Letofsky, and W. Lancee, "Help for Families of Suicide: Survivors Support Program," *Canadian Journal of Psychiatry* 27 (1982): 444-449.

[20] M. Vachon, W. Lyall, J. Rogers, K. Freedman-Letovsky, and S. Freeman, "A Controlled Study of Self-Help Intervention for Widows," *American Journal of Psychiatry*, 137 (1980): 1380-1384; M. Vachon, J. Rogers, W. Lyall, W. Lancee, A. Sheldon, and S. Freeman, "Predictors and Correlates of Adaptation to Conjugal Bereavement," *American Journal of Psychiatry* 139 (1982): 998-1002; M. Vachon, A. Sheldon, W. Lancee, W. Lyall, J. Rogers, and S. Freeman, "Correlates of Enduring Distress Patterns Following Bereavement: Social Network, Life Situation, and Personality," *Psychological Medicine* 12 (1982): 783-788.

[21] A. Beck, *Depression: Causes and Treatment* (Philadelphia: University of Pennsylvania Press, 1972).

[22] M. Hamilton, "A Rating Scale for Depression." *Journal of Neurology, Neurosurgery, and Psychiatry* 23 (1960): 56-66.

[23] W. Zung, "A Self Rating Depression Scale," *Archives of General Psychiatry* 12 (January 1965): 64.

[24] C. Saunders and P. Mauger, *A Manual for the Grief Experience Inventory* (Tampa: University of South Florida, 1979).

[25] T. Fauschingbaur, R. DeVaul, and S. Zisook, "Development of the Texas Inventory of Grief," *American Journal of Psychiatry* 134 (1977): 696-699.

[26] B. Singh and B. Raphael, "Postdisaster Morbidity of the Bereaved: A Possible Role for Preventive Psychiatry," *Journal of Nervous and Mental Disease* 169 (1981): 203-212.

[27] A. Demi and M. Schroeder, "Psychometric Evaluation of a Bereavement Instrument," 1984 (unpublished paper).

[28] R. C. Aitken, "Assessment of Mood by Analogue," in A. Beck, H. Resnick, and D. Lattieri (eds.), *Prediction of Suicide* (Bowie, Md.: Charles Press, 1974).

[29] Joint Commission on Accreditation of Hospitals (JCAH), *Hospice Standards Manual* (Chicago: JCAH, 1983); JCAH, *Hospice Self-Assessment and Survey Guide* (Chicago: JCAH, 1983).

[30] JCAH, *Self-Assessment Guide,* pp. 15-16.

[31] *Ibid.,* pp. 16-17.

REFERENCES

Aitken, R. C. "Assessment of Mood by Analogue." In A. Beck, H. Resnick, and D. Lattieri, *Prediction of Suicide.* Bowie, Md: Charles Press, 1974.

Ball, J. F. "Widow's Grief: Impact of Age and Mode of Death." *Omega: Journal of Death and Dying* 8 (1977): 307-333.

Beck, A. *Depression: Causes and Treatment.* Philadelphia: University of Pennsylvania Press, 1972.

Caplan, G. *Principles of Preventive Psychiatry.* New York: Basic Books, 1964.

_____. "Foreword." In I. Glick, R. Weiss, and C. M. Parkes, *The First Year of Bereavement.* New York: John Wiley & Sons, 1974.

Clayton, P. "The Clinical Morbidity of the First Year of Bereavement: A Review." *Comprehensive Psychiatry* 14 (1973): 151-157.

Demi, A. "Adjustment to Widowhood After a Sudden Death: Suicide and Non-Suicide Survivors Compared." In M. Batey (ed.), *Communicating Nursing Research.* Boulder, Colo.: WICHE, 1978.

_____. "Mental Health of Widows After a Sudden Death: Suicide and Non-Suicide Survivors Compared." *Proceedings of the Tenth International Congress for Suicide Prevention and Crisis Intervention,* Ottawa, Canada, 1979.

_____. *Bereavement Support Groups: Leadership Manual.* Denver, Colo.: Grief Education Institute, 1981.

_____. "Social Adjustment of Widows After a Sudden Death: Suicide and Non-Suicide Survivors Compared." *Death Education,* in press.

Demi, A. and M. A. Schroeder. "Psychometric Evaluation of a Bereavement Instrument." 1984 (Unpublished paper).

Derogatis, L., R. Lipman, K. Rickels, E. Uhlenhuth, and L. Covi. "The Hopkins Symptom Checklist (HSCL): A Self-Report Symptom Inventory." *Behavioral Science* 19 (1974): 1-15.

Epstein, G., L. Weitz, H. Roback, and E. McKee. "Research on Bereavement: A Selective and Critical Review." *Comprehensive Psychiatry* 16 (1975): 537-546.

Fauschingbaur, T., R. DeVaul, and S. Zisook. "Development of the Texas Inventory of Grief." *American Journal of Psychiatry* 134 (1977): 696-699.

Fulton, R., and D. Gottesman. "Anticipatory Grief: A Psychosocial Concept Reconsidered." *British Journal of Psychiatry* 137 (1980): 45-54.

Gerber, I., R. Rusalem, N. Hannon, D. Batten, and A. Arkin. "Anticipatory Grief and Aged Widows and Widowers." *Journal of Gerontology* 30 (1974): 225-229.

Glick, R., R. Weiss, and C. Parkes. *The First Year of Bereavement*. New York: John Wiley & Sons, 1974.

Goldberg, D. "The Detection of Psychiatric Illness by Questionnaire." *British Journal of Psychiatry* 129 (1976): 61-67.

Hamilton, M. "A Rating Scale for Depression." *Journal of Neurology, Neurosurgery, and Psychiatry* 23 (1960): 56-66.

Health Care Financing Administration. *Federal Register*, August 22, 1983.

International Work Group on Death, Dying and Bereavement. "Assumptions and Principles Underlying Standards for Terminal Care." *American Journal of Nursing*, February 1979, pp. 296-297.

Joint Commission on Accreditation of Hospitals (JCAH). *Hospice Self-Assessment and Survey Guide*. Chicago, Ill.: Joint Commission on Accreditation of Hospitals, 1983.

_____. *Hospice Standards Manual*. Chicago, Ill.: Joint Commission on Accreditation of Hospitals, 1983.

Kraus, A., and A. Lilienfeld. "Some Epidemiologic Aspects of the High Mortality Rate in the Young Widowed Group." *Journal of Chronic Disease* (1959): 207-217.

Lack, S. *Philosophy and Organization of a Hospice Program*. New Haven, Conn.: Hospice of New Haven, 1978.

Lindemann, E. "Symptomatology and Management of Acute Grief." *American Journal of Psychiatry* 101 (1944): 141-148.

Lindstrom, B. "Operating a Hospice Bereavement Program." In C. Corr and D. Corr (eds.), *Hospice Care: Principles and Practices*. New York: Springer, 1983.

Maddison, A., and A. Viola. "The Health of Widows in the Year Following Bereavement." *Journal of Psychosomatic Research* 12 (1968): 297-306.

Murphy, S. "After Mount St. Helens: Disaster Stress Research." *Journal of Psychosocial Nursing and Mental Health Services* 22 (July 1984): 8-18.

Parkes, C. M. "The Effects of Bereavement on Physical and Mental Health: A Study of the Case Records of Widows." *British Medical Journal* 2 (1964): 274-280.

_____. "Determinants of Outcome Following Bereavement." *Omega: Journal of Death and Dying* 6 (1975): 302-323.

Parkes, C. M., and R. Weiss. *Recovery from Bereavement*. New York: Basic Books, 1983.

Quayhagen, M., and A. Demi. "Bereavement and Aging, Ethnic and Sex Differences: A Pilot Study." Unpublished paper, 1979.

Rogers, J., A. Sheldon, C. Barwick, K. Letofsky, and W. Lancee. "Help for Families of Suicide: Survivors Support Systems." *Canadian Journal of Psychiatry* 27 (1982): 444-449.

Saunders, C., and P. Mauger. *A Manual for the Grief Experience Inventory.* Tampa: University of South Florida, 1979.

Schoenberg, B., A. Carr, A. Kutscher, D. Peretz, and I. Goldberg (eds.). *Anticipatory Grief.* New York: Columbia University Press, 1974.

Singh, B., and B. Raphael. "Postdisaster Morbidity of the Bereaved: A Possible Role for Preventive Psychiatry." *Journal of Nervous and Mental Disease* 169 (1981): 203-212.

Vachon, M., W. Lyall, J. Rogers, K. Freedman-Letovsky, and S. Freeman. "A Controlled Study of Self-Help Intervention for Widows." *American Journal of Psychiatry* 137 (1980): 1380-1384.

Vachon, M., J. Rogers, W. Lyall, W. Lancee, A. Sheldon, and S. Freeman. "Predictors and Correlates of Adaptation to Conjugal Bereavement." *American Journal of Psychiatry* 139 (1982): 998-1002.

Vachon, M., A. Sheldon, W. Lancee, W. Lyall, J. Rogers, and S. Freeman. "Correlates of Enduring Distress Patterns Following Bereavement: Social Network, Life Situation and Personality." *Psychological Medicine* 12 (1982): 783-788.

Volkan, V. "The Linking Objects of Pathological Mourners." *Archives of General Psychiatry* 27 (1972): 215-221.

Volkan, V. "Typical Findings in Pathologic Grief." *Psychiatric Quarterly* 44 (1970): 231-250.

Worden, J. *Grief Counseling and Grief Therapy.* New York: Springer, 1982.

Zung, W. "A Self Rating Depression Scale." *Archives of General Psychiatry* 12 (January 1965): 64.

Chapter 9

Current Issues and Future Directions

Jessie F. Igou

Hospice philosophy emphasizes helping a dying person to live fully or optimally during a time of decline. As hospice undergoes a transitional period and moves beyond the initial stage of development, it seems an appropriate time to review current issues that face hospice programs and to clarify these issues in order to provide direction for the future. Various authors would identify different issues, but I suggest that at this time hospice programs should consider issues related to (1) the nature and scope of practice with dying patients, (2) the nature and scope of practice with their families, (3) the needs of staff members who care for these individuals, and (4) research. The remainder of this chapter addresses each of these issues.

NATURE AND SCOPE OF PRACTICE WITH HOSPICE PATIENTS

A human being is a complex and integrated being. The quality of a person's life represents the interaction of the physical, psychological, sociological, and spiritual components. Any condition or disease affects not only the body but also the mind and the spirit. For this reason, a holistic approach to the care of an ill person and his or her family is important. Holism is a concept of total nurturing with an emphasis on care. This approach appears essential to caring for dying patients in a hospice program since this is a time when the physical, emotional, and spiritual needs of patients and families are greatest. A holistic view does not see any dimension or component of a person as being optimal or peripheral but instead sees the person as a totality with needs in each sphere. If a change in one dimension occurs, the total system is affected. If one dimension is neglected, all components are diminished. Although integration of mind and body is not a new idea, and although hospice philosophy incorporates holism, this approach has not always been followed clinically, as caregivers often focus on physical needs while other needs are viewed peripherally and therefore go unmet.[1]

It seems that it is time to expand the nature and scope of practice for hospice caregivers to include more therapeutic modalities, both traditional and nontraditional. Those modalities that promote holism can be employed in conjunction with traditional medical treatment. Hospice caregivers should not be expected to be experts in all these modalities, but they should be aware of a variety of methods so that they can guide the patient and family in finding sources of help and support.

Travis[2] has developed a wellness model that focuses on being aware and taking care of the body, self, and mind. In this model, all three components overlap, are closely affected by one another, and are united by self-responsibility. Wellness is enhanced by a growth-promoting, supportive environment, the kind of environment that should be provided by a hospice program. A modification of the Travis model in which the dimension of mind replaces the dimension of self could be useful as a holistic framework for approaching the dying patient and family. Integration of physical, emotional, and spiritual needs is a part of this model and would provide direction for caregivers.

According to Pelletier,[3] a holistic approach to health has six characteristics, three of which are that (1) each person must be seen as unique and represents an interaction of body, mind, and spirit, (2) the health care provider must come to know himself or herself, and (3) health care is not limited to traditional medical regimes. The first and last characteristics provide the basis for using an array of traditional and nontraditional modalities to meet needs in a human being's three integrated spheres. It may be necessary for caregivers of dying patients to become familiar with both Eastern and Western traditions and the therapies that each has to offer. Some of the nontraditional therapies can be used to overcome fears and negative feelings experienced by patients and families.

Physiological Dimension

Physiological fears or threats that patients with a diagnosis of cancer experience are pain; loss of strength; loss of skin integrity; aversive responses to medical therapies, such as nausea and vomiting; and loss of nutritional and hydration status. The usual interventions are related to relieving pain and managing symptoms by medication administration, caring for the skin, helping to conserve energy, and managing nutritional intake. In addition, other modalities may be used to enhance control of the body, including autogenic training, progressive muscle relaxation training, biofeedback, self-hypnosis, and therapeutic touch.

Autogenic training is a deep relaxation technique based on passive attention to the body developed by Shultz in 1932.[4] Shultz combined the concept of self-hypnosis with a series of six exercises designed to integrate mental and physical functions and to include states of deep physiological and mental relaxation. The exercises are practiced in a quiet atmosphere, with the patient in a horizontal position with closed eyes. Exercise 1 induces sensations of heaviness of the limbs, while exercise 2 induces sensations of warmth in the limbs. Exercises 3 and 4 deal with cardiac and respiratory regulation, respectively. Exercise 5 induces a feeling of warmth in the upper abdomen, and exercise 6 induces a sense of coolness in the forehead. Autogenic training appears to be an effective technique for controlling pain and anxiety in cancer patients.

Progressive muscle relaxation training, developed by Jacobson in 1928, can also be used to combat physical pain or anxiety.[5] It is a technique for achieving discriminatory control over skeletal muscles until low levels of tonus are achieved in large muscle groups.[6] The patient learns to tense and relax various muscle groups in the body sequentially. At the same time, one allows one's attention to drift to the feelings associated with relaxation and tension. This technique has been effectively used in the treatment of a variety of problems, including headaches, insomnia, anxiety, and hypertension. In cancer patients, aversive reactions to chemotherapy have been significantly reduced in individuals who have practiced muscle relaxation and guided imagery. Patients who use relaxation training are reported to be less anxious and nauseated during the chemotherapeutic regime. It is proposed that the conscious muscle relaxation and guided imagery function as cognitive distractors and serve to help patients focus on pleasant thoughts rather than on worry, pain, and sickness.[7]

Biofeedback is another technique that can be used to help patients become aware of and gain control over one or more involuntary body functions and responses. Through electronic sensing, the biofeedback machine gives the patient information about himself to help him learn to control physical, mental, or emotional processes. Biofeedback has been found to help decrease chronic pain in cancer patients by training the patient to shift attention away from the pain to a different inner feeling. This alpha feedback technique can also be combined with hypnosis, which produces a relaxation that has been shown to be effective in reducing pain in 50 percent of patients.[8] Biofeedback is best used as a way to relax, reduce anxiety, and get in touch with the inner self.

Self-hypnosis is another modality that can be used to attain conscious control over the body as well as the mind. The results are better management of stress and pain. Because it is a learned skill, it can be used daily by dying patients, family members, or staff to keep in touch with themselves and maintain some control over their physical and emotional symptoms.

Therapeutic touch, when done consciously by centering (the healer consciously quieting his or her own mind), with compassion and intention (intent of the healer to help), has been identified as one of the most effective therapeutic modalities for the dying person. Fanslow states that "the act of therapeutic touch consists of centering, assessment and energy transfer,"[9] or making energy available. Dying patients are often more receptive and open to this energy than are other patients. A physiological effect of therapeutic touch is profound relaxation, which appears to be heightened in the dying person, and decreased pain.

Psychological and spiritual effects of this type of therapy include enhancement of a loving, caring relationship between patient and caregiver and attainment of an inner sense of peace and calm and a harmonious inner balance. The energy that is transferred from helper to patient helps the dying person to let go and makes the anticipatory phase of dying much more tranquil. Results of several research studies support the possibility that touch has a calming and comforting effect on seriously ill patients[10] and can significantly reduce anxiety in hospital patients.[11] It appears that dying patients who have experienced therapeutic touch have less pain and an enhanced feeling of well-being, indicating that this modality should be considered an important adjunct to other therapies for the hospice patient. Although touch has been recognized for centuries as a therapeutic technique, it is not universally accepted by caregivers.

Therapeutic touch also appears to be an effective means of helping family members and caregivers let go.[12] As they observe the dying person's transformation to a sense of inner peace, they can release the bonds that hold them to the dying person.

Emotional Dimension

A holistic approach to dying patients in a hospice program dictates that patients' and families' emotional or psychological needs must be attended to. Nowhere are emotional needs as urgent as for dying patients. Their most common fears include fear of pain, addiction to pain-relieving medications, financial insecurity, fear of many and various losses including loss of independence, loss of sexuality, loss of dignity, and loss of future plans. Three other major threats to the dying person are (1) loss of control or a sense of powerlessness and inability to control body functions, life-style choices, and environment, (2) changes in body image which may result in loss of self-esteem and altered self-concept, and (3) loneliness and isolation. For most dying patients, the fear of separation from significant others supersedes the fear of physical pain. Dr. Nancy Nichols, founder of the hospice program at Baltimore's Union Memorial Hospital, claims, "The most overwhelming emotion for many patients is fear of abandonment."[13]

A study conducted by Nash showed that self-esteem needs were a great issue for 24 terminally ill adults.[14] Ninety percent of the respondents indicated feeling a lack of dignity. The patients' behavioral responses showed feelings of powerlessness, loneliness, pain, and difficulty coping with multiple losses. Nash states that "the fulfillment of a person's biological needs is definable and concrete. However, the characteristics which make him human—his relatedness and feelings—are much more abstract, less concrete, and more difficult of definition. Yet it is the resolution of these needs which essentially gives meaning to life."[15]

The goal of the hospice caregiver is to facilitate peaceful acceptance of inevitable death, or at least to allow the patient the opportunity to communicate his feelings. Four techniques to facilitate communication and thus enhance emotional integrity are: (1) using the journalistic style of questioning, (2) active listening and empathizing, (3) touching, and (4) facilitating the life-review process.[16] The journalistic style of questioning helps guide the patient in problem solving. Active listening and empathy must also be used in working with a dying patient; this requires the caregiver to try to see the patient's world from the patient's point of view. The value of therapeutic touch was mentioned earlier as a way of decreasing emotional distance between the patient and the caregiver, thus enhancing communication and peaceful acceptance of death by the dying person.

Facilitating the life-review process is also a therapeutic modality that can be extremely supportive to the dying person. This process allows the patient to review past relationships and stressful events. By engaging in the review, "patients are able to maintain power over themselves, and opportunities to psychologically make things right and prepare for impending loss of life are opened."[17] Life review helps the dying person meet some of the psychological threats of loss of control and power.

Any technique that helps the patient feel that he has some measure of control over his life and allows him to express his fears and concerns will be of emotional benefit. Various traditional and nontraditional modalities can be used to enhance psychological wellness in dying patients and their family members. Those mentioned under the physiological dimension—autogenic training, progressive relaxation, biofeedback, self-hypnosis, and therapeutic touch—can also be used to attend to emotional needs. These methods can help lessen anxiety and generate feelings of peace and harmony. Other methods, such as facilitative communication strategies and life review, will enhance the dying patient's sense of control and self-esteem.

Spiritual Dimension

Unmet spiritual needs or concerns can be a source of fear, pain, and isolation for patients. Although spiritual well-being is recognized to be as important as physiological and emotional well-being, this dimension is often sidelined by caregivers.

A critical distinction needs to be made between religious and spiritual needs. Dewey defines religion as a belief in God or a higher being than man,[18] whereas spiritual well-being has been defined as the "affirmation of life in a relationship with God, self, community and environment that nurtures and celebrates wholeness."[19] Spiritual well-being goes beyond the exclusively religious domain; it pertains to "intangible, nonmaterial characteristics, needs, or qualities which all human beings possess."[20] The 1981 White House Conference on Spiritual Well-Being concluded "that all [persons] are 'spiritual' even if they have no use for religious institutions and practice no personal piety."[21] Dewey suggests that those who have no faith in God also need to be accepted and comforted.[22] Patients need to know that they will not be alone. Thus addressing the spiritual needs of a dying hospice patient and his family means attending to religious needs in a specific sense and spiritual needs in a general sense. Acknowledging and helping the dying person to acknowledge his or her own spiritual nature can help give the remaining period of life its fullest meaning. If caregivers can recognize the spiritual needs of the dying person, they can then assist him in meeting those needs and enhancing a sense of wholeness.

The hospice caregiver's responsibility is to assess the spiritual needs of the patient and the family. The assessment process and the planned interventions should provide a forum for the patient to express his feelings. This aspect of care can be given by the hospice nurse, who might also make a referral to a clergyman, if the patient desires. It is most important to see that the patient has someone to talk to. Dewey states that some dying individuals fear pain and body image changes, and may lose a sense of self-importance.[23] During these times, they may find it difficult or impossible to pray and thus feel guilty because they lack religious fervor. Dewey concludes that it is not useful to talk a lot about God but helpful to listen to patients and families as they identify their concerns and fears. The caregiver should encourage the patient to express feelings of guilt, anger, and isolation. The dying need help in understanding their anger and need to feel accepted even though they are angry with God.

For hospice caregivers to provide spiritual support, they must be willing to spend time with patients—time to help them feel loved and important, and time to share a sense of hope. Dewey sums up how best to meet the spiritual needs of dying patients by her statement that "patients need to know that they will not be alone. What is essential is that our behavior be loving toward all people and that it convey a sense of worth, dignity, and respect for the value of every individual."[24]

In addition to working with individual patients and families in the hospice program, caregivers should work with the religious community to help develop and promote groups such as the Los Angeles Jewish Hospice Commission, which was organized to explain and promote the hospice concept throughout the Jewish community and to promote understanding of the teachings of the Jewish religion relative to the care of the terminally ill patient and his or her family.[25] This model might serve to guide other religious groups to organize within their community so that dying individuals can be cared for within the precepts of their own faith. This would be one step in ensuring that psychological and spiritual needs are met in dying persons.

Therapeutic modalities are described in the literature that can be used to enhance spiritual wellness. Inner dialogue is one such modality. This concept, based on the idea that each person has an intuitive knowledge of how to exist in peace, offers the opportunity to bridge the gap between mind and body.[26] Inner dialogue allows patients to search for symptoms of disharmony that prevent them from functioning optimally. It takes the patient out of the passive role and into an active, responsible role.

There are different ways to get in touch with this intuitive knowledge. One method is to have a dialogue with an archetypal figure to learn what existing symptoms mean and find ways to relieve them. The body is viewed as the battleground for conflicting attitudes that resolve themselves once the person is able to talk about the conflict. Another way to have an inner dialogue is to learn to imagine an inner advisor in a shape or form that seems helpful. The advisor should have qualities that are helpful to the patient, and it is important that the patient be honest with the advisor. Once the dialogue is completed, the patient should be able to exist in peace.[26]

Another modality that can promote spiritual, psychological, and physiological well-being is the practice of yoga, which is defined by Weller as a means of self-discovery, self-discipline, and self-improvement. She lists the components of yoga as physical and breathing exercises as well as concentration, meditation, and relaxation techniques.[27]

While the asanas (postures or exercises) might not be possible for the dying person, family or staff mights might utilize these to promote health of the spinal column, spinal nerves, muscles, and overall general health. The pranayama, or breathing control exercises, on the other hand, can be used by family, staff, and dying patients to fight the effects of tension. Shallow, irregular respiration can lead to anxiety and restlessness, while smooth, regular breathing has a calming influence on the mind.[28]

Yoga also involves concentration and meditation techniques. Yoga concentration techniques train the person to direct attention on one activity and hold it, to the exclusion of all else. Weller states, "One learns to control circumstances, rather than be at their mercy."[29]

Yoga meditation techniques progress naturally from the concentration exercises. They require physical and mental stillness for anywhere from 10 to 20 or more minutes at a time. Yoga relaxation techniques can be either local or systemic. In the former, the person learns to eliminate tension from a specific body part, while in the latter, the entire organism is taught to relax. It appears that spiritual and psychological benefits may be attained from the practice of yoga, including attainment of an internal state of control, balance, harmony, and peace.

Other activities, such as a daily ritual, can enhance spiritual wellness in patients, families, and staff. Schiff, after losing a son, felt that having a disciplined, systematic routine of going to the temple every evening for a period of time made her face the truth daily and made her go through the grieving process more gently and quickly than she might otherwise. She recommends setting aside 10 minutes a day to think deeply and suggests that this can be done even if the person's faith offers no religious service or the person chooses not to partake in one.[30]

The essence of hospice seems to be found in the spiritual dimension. Hospice caregivers must assure patients that they will not be forsaken but will be surrounded by loved ones and friends, will have their pain relieved, and will be treated with love and grace in order to arrive at spiritual peace.

NATURE AND SCOPE OF PRACTICE WITH HOSPICE FAMILIES

Toynbee has made the assertion that, typically, death is a dyadic event:

> The two-sidedness of death is a fundamental feature of death . . . the sting of death is less sharp for the person who dies than it is for the bereaved survivor . . . . There are two parties to the suffering that death inflicts; and in the apportionment of this suffering, the survivor takes the brunt.[31]

Shneidman more recently proposed that the survivor is the victim and that he eventually becomes the patient if he is not helped through the grieving process.[32] He has developed the concept of postvention, or working with survivors, and suggests that this should be an integral part of the health care system.

Traditionally, the family has been expected to be the primary source of support to the family member who is dying or undergoing any major crisis. Recently, the nuclear family has been viewed not merely as the major source of refuge and protection for the dying person but actually as the unit facing the disease and crisis.[33] A diagnosis of cancer not only disrupts the life of the dying person but also threatens the functioning and integrity of the family system. Caregivers must offer support and assistance to the individual family members and to the family unit as a whole.

If family members are not helped to cope with the dying of a loved one, lowered self-esteem and self-worth, self-confidence, and security may result. Positive coping patterns and a good social support system can mitigate a crisis.[34] The reaction of each family member must be assessed and the data used to develop appropriate interventions which will aid the family in their adaptation to the death of a loved one and strengthen the autonomy of each family member. A conceptual approach based on holism, addressing all three dimensions and the needs identified in each, can be utilized by the caregiver in working with individual family members as well as with the dying patient. Biofeedback, autogenic training, relaxation techniques, therapeutic touch, yoga, and meditation can be used by these individuals to relieve anxiety, promote relaxation, enhance a sense of control over their own bodies, and create a sense of balance in their lives.

It is important for caregivers to view the family as a unit of care and to offer care to this unit. In working with families who faced a diagnosis of cancer, Giacquinta developed a model that focuses on 10 phases within four stages that family units go through as a loved one is dying and after the death has occurred. The model is based on interviews with 100 families who described the difficult situations and tasks they encountered during this crisis time. The four stages Giacquinta describes are Living with Cancer, Restructuring in the Living-Dying Interval, Bereavement, and Reestablishment.[35] The model is useful for both assessing the family's needs during the crises and for deciding on interventions to meet those needs.

During the Living with Cancer stage, the family unit becomes aware of the diagnosis and responds with shock and bewilderment. This first phase has been labeled the impact phase. Psychological disturbances, such as insomnia and anorexia, are common, as are psychological distress, despair, and depression. Hospice caregivers must have as their goal the overcoming of this despair and depression by the fostering of hope, helping the family to realize that they can live with the diagnosis, and providing assurance that resources will be available. "Hope cannot be sustained without the support of significant others; it must be generated in the family."[36] The hospice caregiver should encourage hope in both the dying person and the family unit.

The second phase of the Living with Cancer stage, as identified by Giacquinta, is the functional disruption phase. At this time, responsibilities to the dying person supersede responsibilities of household and family management. The major task in this phase is to prevent isolation of family members from one another by encouraging and facilitating communication, cooperation, support, and identification of needs and resources. These actions on the part of the health care giver should foster a sense of cohesion and stability within the family unit.

The third phase in the Living with Cancer stage reflects a search for meaning as members attempt to learn about the diagnosis of cancer and thereby gain mastery over events. There is also an attempt to gain reassurance that other family members will not be affected with the same condition. During this phase, family members become vulnerable to fusion and identification with the dying person. Caregivers should support family members to enable them to maintain their own individual integrity and identity, thus fostering security for the family system.

In the fourth phase in stage 1, informing others, hospice caregivers must foster courage to cope within the family unit by helping individuals communicate internally, gather knowledge, and identify priorities for action.

The final phase in the Living with Cancer stage is a time when emotions may become volatile and erratic as family members fear losing control. Loss of control does not occcur, however, if people acknowledge and express their emotions. As family members lose control, they can be overwhelmed by a sense of helplessness. During this phase, caregivers should foster the family members' problem-solving skills in order to decrease the sense of helplessness.

When the individual who is dying of cancer relinquishes functional and familial roles, the family enters the Restructuring in the Living-Dying Interval stage. The two phases of this stage are reorganization of roles within the family unit and framing of memories, or attempting to remember what the ill family member was like before the diagnosis of cancer. As the family members attempt to take on new roles and establish new rules, hospice caregivers must help prevent competition and foster cooperation. Families are encouraged to recollect their loved one in earlier days through the sharing of stories and pictures.

Stage 3 of the Giacquinta model, Bereavement, is the stage in which separation and mourning occur. During the separation phase, the loved one may lose consciousness and the family begins to sense their overwhelming loss. At this time, caregivers should promote intimacy within the family unit. During this mourning stage, guilt is a major hurdle for the family, and they should be helped to share their feelings about the guilt and their loss.

The final stage in the Giacquinta model is Reestablishment, in which expanding the social network is the last phase. Caregivers should help prevent the family from becoming alienated by encouraging relatedness within the family. "As families become closer and expand their social network, they begin to accept that the death in the family was inevitable but not insurmountable."[37]

MEETING THE NEEDS OF HOSPICE STAFF

As the philosophy of care for the terminally ill has begun to change to a palliative approach that includes physical, psychosocial, and spiritual concerns, caregivers have begun to experience considerable stress. Hospice caregivers give of themselves emotionally over a prolonged period of time without being replenished. Vachon suggests that ultimately they will be psychologically depleted and will have nothing left to give.[38] This "burnout" syndrome results from protracted stress in the occupational setting and occurs in caregivers who are strongly committed to their work rather than to those who are dissatisfied.

The stress that causes burnout can result from organizational factors (schedules, workload, agency conflict), individual factors (personal characteristics of caregivers), and societal factors (cultural and societal characteristics).[39] Vachon observes that caregivers also experience stress when (1) they cannot accept that patients' symptoms cannot be controlled, (2) they work with families whose energies have been drained, (3) they become overinvolved with patients and families and cannot set limits of care, or (4) the patient does not die a "good death."[40]

Freudenberger categorized symptoms and professional burnout into three categories: somatic, interpersonal, and psychological.[41] The somatic symptoms most often include fatigue, gastrointestinal problems, headaches, insomnia, and shortness of breath. The interpersonal symptoms primarily include distancing behaviors, such as avoidance of patients, and acting-out behaviors, such as use of alcohol. Psychological symptoms include anxiety, depression (caused by constant exposure to death), negativism, and unresolved sorrow.[42]

Shneidman suggests that a special in-depth relationship develops between the hospice caregiver and the dying person.[43] He states that because of the intensity of this relationship and the special feelings between these two, when the patient dies the caregiver grieves and might be expected to feel anguish and a great sense of loss.

Suggestions for dealing with stress are based on the premise that mediating factors, such as sense of control of the situation, type and number of coping mechanisms used, and availability of support systems, will influence the hospice caregiver's response to the stressful situation. While caregivers may not be able to control the dying patient's diagnosis and course of illness, they can utilize some of the previously discussed stress-reduction techniques, such as biofeedback, relaxation techniques, yoga, and meditation. Relaxation, yoga, and meditation techniques can be practiced in a quiet spot for a short period of time, allowing the caregiver to relax physically and free the mind to cope with other stressors.

The hospice caregiver should have a well-integrated social support system within and outside the hospice. This can be provided through hospice team support meetings, continuing peer and supervisory support, and consultation with mental health professionals. This support system will provide a forum for ventilation and sharing of feelings.

Changes in working conditions can also help reduce staff stress. A variety of work patterns should be tried in an effort to discover optimal assignment patterns. Also, time might be made available to the staff to practice some of the relaxation techniques or participate in support groups.

It is important that the staff and the administration in a hospice unit be able to recognize early signs of emotional exhaustion and burnout. Appropriate steps can then be taken by the caregiver, and supportive care can be offered by the agency. However, it appears much more valuable and humane to prevent emotional exhaustion from occurring. A holistic approach focusing on the physical, emotional, and spiritual needs of caregivers should be practiced by the caregivers themselves and by the employing agency.

RESEARCH

The last major issue is that of research. Since hospice is a recent phenomenon, few qualitative studies that evaluate the clinical effectiveness and cost effectiveness of hospice care have been completed.

Clinical Effectiveness

There are numerous questions about clinical effectiveness that have not yet been answered and that deserve attention. We need to search for and test new methods for relieving physiological, psychological, and spiritual pain and for evaluating the effectiveness of methods already in use. Methods for fostering family stability, family cohesion, and family control need to be developed. Questions related to staff burnout, such as what kind of person is likely to suffer from emotional exhaustion and what kinds of organizations or jobs predispose caregivers to burnout, should be addressed. Patients, families, and staff members should be studied in order to determine their views of what their needs are, rather than providing care according to the caregiver's or agency's perceptions. Also, high-risk hospice patients and families should be identified so that special attention can be focused on them.

Overall, research needs to be completed to determine if hospice care is "better," is more therapeutically effective, and results in more positive outcomes such as enhanced physical, emotional, and spiritual states than nonhospice care.

Cost Effectiveness

The second major research thrust should be made to determine whether hospice care is cost effective. While it may be a more humane, holistic way to care for dying individuals, what are the cost implications of hospice? Preliminary studies suggest that hospice may be less expensive than conventional care.[44] In this day of financial cutbacks, and in anticipation of reimbursement for hospice care, caregivers and researchers must carry out more studies on cost effectiveness. Governmental agencies as well as private agencies want to know not only what their money is buying but whether the services they are purchasing are cost effective.

SUMMARY

Hospice care is a relatively new approach to care in the United States. Now that hospice is being integrated into the health care system, it is appropriate to identify the major issues facing hospice. Although many issues have become apparent over the last decade, it seems important to reassess the scope and nature of the care offered by hospice caregivers to both patients and their families. The issue of professional burnout continues to be a critical one since empirical studies suggest that the incidence of burnout is still high in caregivers who invest large amounts of emotional energy in their work. Therapeutic and holistic methods of prevention and treatment of staff burnout must be found and utilized. Research is the vehicle through which needs of patients, families, and staff can be identified and new therapies developed and evaluated for their clinical effectiveness. In addition, the cost effectiveness of hospice must be determined if this holistic, nurturing approach to care for the dying is to survive the next decade.

NOTES

[1] Joan Luckman and Karen C. Sorensen, *Medical-Surgical Nursing: A Psychophysiologic Approach* (Philadelphia: Saunders, 1980), pp. 26, 70.

[2] John Travis, *Wellness Workbook for Helping Professionals* (Mill Valley, Calif.: Wellness Associates, 1981), p. 100.

[3] Kenneth R. Pelletier, *Mind as Healer, Mind as Slayer* (New York: Dell, 1977), pp. 230, 318, 319.

[4] Luckman and Sorensen, *op. cit.,* p. 70.

[5] *Ibid.*

[6] Judith M. Richter and Rebecca Sloan, "A Relaxation Technique," *American Journal of Nursing,* November 1979, pp. 1960-1964.

[7] Jeanne N. Lyles, Thomas G. Burish, Mary G. Krozely, and Robert K. Oldham, "Efficacy of Relaxation Training and Guided Imagery in Reducing the Adversiveness of Cancer Chemotherapy," *Journal of Consulting and Clinical Psychology* 50 (1982): 509-524.

[8] Barbara B. Brown, *Stress and the Art of Biofeedback* (New York: Harper & Row, 1977), p. 168.

[9] Cathleen A. Fanslow, "Therapeutic Touch: A Healing Modality Throughout Life," *Topics in Clinical Nursing,* July 1983, pp. 72-79.

[10] Ruth McCorkle, "Effects of Touch on Seriously Ill Patients," *Nursing Research* 23 (March-April 1974): 125-132.

[11] Patricia Heidt, "Effect of Therapeutic Touch on Anxiety Level of Hospitalized Patients," *Nursing Research* 30 (January-February 1981): 32-37.

[12] Fanslow, *op. cit.*

[13] *Johns Hopkins Magazine (Hopkins News)* 25 (June 1984): 53.

[14] Mary L. Nash, "Dignity of Person in the Final Phase of Life—An Exploratory Study," *Omega* 8 (1977): 71, 72, 79.

[15] *Ibid.,* p. 72.

[16] Noreen D. Cerino, "Therapeutic Communication: A Necessity in Hospice Care," *The American Journal of Hospice Care,* 1 (Spring 1984): 21.

[17] *Ibid.,* p. 23.

[18] Darlene Dewey, "Function of Religion in Clinical Practice," in *Current Perspectives in Oncologic Nursing* (Vol. 2), ed. Carolyn Kellogg and Barbara Sullivan (St. Louis: Mosby, 1978), pp. 151-153.

[19] National Interfaith Coalition on Aging, *Spiritual Well-Being: A Definition,* 1975. (One-page definition and commentary.)

[20] White House Conference on Aging, *Executive Summary of Technical Committee on Creating an Age Integrated Society: Implications for Spiritual Well-Being* (Washington, D.C.: U.S. Government Printing Office, 1981), p. 3.

[21] David O. Moberg, *Spiritual Well-Being: Background and Issues of the Technical Committee on Spiritual Well-Being,* 1971 White House Conference on Aging (Washington, D.C.: U.S. Government Printing Office), p. 3.

[22] Dewey, *op. cit.*

[23] *Ibid.*

[24] *Ibid.,* p. 153.

[25] Audrey P. Harris, "Report: Los Angeles Jewish Hospice Commission," *The American Journal of Hospice Care* 1 (Spring 1984): 24-25.

[26] Carolyn C. Clark, "Inner Dialogue: A Self-Healing Approach for Nurses and Clients," *American Journal of Nursing,* June 1981, pp. 1191-1193.

[27] Stella Weller, "Unending Thoughts," *Nursing Mirror,* April 30, 1981, pp. 20-22.

[28] *Ibid.*

[29] *Ibid.,* p. 21.

[30] Harriet S. Schiff, *The Bereaved Parent* (New York: Penguin, 1978), p. 115.

[31] Arnold Toynbee, A. Keith Mant, Ninian Smart, John Hinton, Simon Yudkin, Eric Rhode, Rosalind Heywood, and H. H. Price, *Man's Concern with Death* (New York: McGraw-Hill, 1969), pp. 267-271.

[32] Edwin S. Shneidman, "Some Aspects of Psychotherapy with Dying Persons," in *Death: Current Perspectives,* ed. E. Shneidman (Palo Alto, Calif.: Mayfield Publishing Co., 1980), pp. 206, 212, 234.

[33] Barbara Giacquinta, "Helping Families Face the Crisis of Cancer," *American Journal of Nursing,* October 1977, pp. 1585-1588.

[34] Imelda Clements, "Stress Adaptation," in *Family Health: A Theoretical Approach to Care,* ed. I. Clements and F. Roberts (New York: John Wiley, 1983), p. 139.

[35] Giacquinta, *op. cit.,* p. 1586.

[36] *Ibid.,* p. 1588.

[37] *Ibid.*

[38] Mary L. Vachon, "Staff Stress in Care of the Terminally Ill," in *Hospice Care: Principles and Practice,* ed. Charles Corr and Donna Corr (New York: Springer Publishing, 1983), pp. 238-241.

[39] Cary Cherniss, *Staff Burnout: Job Stress in the Human Services* (Beverly Hills: Sage, 1980), p. 63.

[40] Vachon, *op. cit.*

[41] Herbert J. Freundenberger, "Burn Out: The Organizational Menace," *Training and Development Journal* 31 (1977): 26-27.

[42] Vachon, "Motivation and Stress Experienced by Staff Working with the Terminally Ill," *Death Education* 2 (1978): 117.

[43] Schneidman, *op. cit.*

[44] Howard G. Birnbaum and David Kidder, "What Does Hospice Cost?" *American Journal of Public Health,* 74(7): 689-697.

REFERENCES

Brown, Barbara B. *Stress and the Art of Biofeedback.* New York: Harper & Row, 1977.

Cerino, Noreen D. "Therapeutic Communications: A Necessity in Hospice Care." *The American Journal of Hospice Care* 1 (Spring 1984): 21.

Cherniss, Cary. *Staff Burnout: Job Stress in the Human Services.* Beverly Hills: Sage Publications, 1980.

Clark, Carolyn C. "Inner Dialogue: A Self-Healing Approach for Nurses and Clients." *American Journal of Nursing,* June 1981, pp. 11, 91, 93.

Clements, Imelda. "Stress Adaptation." In *Family Health: A Theoretical Approach to Care,* ed. I. Clements and F. Roberts. New York: John Wiley, 1983.

Corr, Charles A., and Donna M. Corr. *Hospice Care: Principles and Practice.* New York: Springer Publishing, 1983.

Dewey, Darlene. "Function of Religion in Clinical Practice." In *Current Perspectives in Oncologic Nursing* (Vol. 2), ed. Carolyn Kellogg and Barbara Sullivan. St. Louis: C. V. Mosby, 1978.

Fanslow, Cathleen A. "Therapeutic Touch: A Healing Modality Throughout Life." *Topics in Clinical Nursing,* July 1983, pp. 72-79.

Freundenberger, Herbert J. "Burn Out: The Organizational Menace." *Training and Development Journal* 31 (1977): 26-27.

Giacquinta, Barbara. "Helping Families Face the Crisis of Cancer." *American Journal of Nursing,* October 1977, pp. 1585-1588.

Harris, Audrey P. "Report: Los Angeles Jewish Hospice Commission." *The American Journal of Hospice Care* 1 (Spring 1984): 24-25.

Heidt, Patricia. "Effect of Therapeutic Touch on Anxiety Level of Hospitalized Patients." *Nursing Research* 30 (January-February): 32-37.

Luckman, Joan, and Karen C. Sorensen. *Medical-Surgical Nursing: A Psychophysiologic Approach.* Philadelphia: W. B. Saunders, 1980.

Lyles, Jeanne N., Thomas G. Burish, Mary G. Krozely, and Robert K. Oldham. "Efficacy of Relaxation Training and Guided Imagery in Reducing the Adversiveness of Cancer Chemotherapy." *Journal of Consulting and Clinical Psychology* 50 (1982): 509-524.

McCorkle, Ruth. "Effects of Touch on Seriously Ill Patients." *Nursing Research* 23 (March-April 1974): 125-132.

Moberg, David O. *Spiritual Well-Being: Background and Issues of the Technical Committee on Spiritual Well-Being.* 1971 White House Conference on Aging. Washington, D.C.: U.S. Government Printing Office, 1971.

Nash, Mary L. "Dignity of Person in the Final Phase of Life—An Exploratory Study." *Omega* 8 (1977): 71, 72, 79.

National Interfaith Coalition on Aging. *Spiritual Well-Being: A Definition.* 1975. (One-page definition and commentary.)

Pelletier, Kenneth R. *Mind as Healer, Mind as Slayer.* New York: Dell, 1977.

Richter, Judith M., and Rebecca Sloan. "A Relaxation Technique." *American Journal of Nursing,* November 1979, pp. 1960-1964.

Saunders, Cicely, Dorothy H. Summers, and Neville Teller. *Hospice: The Living Idea.* Philadelphia: W. B. Saunders, 1981.

Schiff, Harriet S. *The Bereaved Parent.* New York: Penguin, 1978.

Shneidman, Edwin S. "Some Aspects of Psychotherapy with Dying Persons." In *Death: Current Perspectives,* ed. E. Shneidman. Palo Alto, Calif.: Mayfield Publishing, 1980.

Stoddard, Sandol. *The Hospice Movement: A Better Way of Caring for the Dying.* Briarcliff Manor, N.Y.: Stein and Day, 1978.

Toynbee, Arnold, A. Keith Mant, Ninian Smart, John Hinton, Simon Yudkin, Eric Rhode, Rosalind Heywood, and H. H. Price. *Man's Concern with Death.* New York: McGraw-Hill, 1969.

Travis, John. *Wellness Workbook for Helping Professionals.* Mill Valley, Calif.: Wellness Associates, 1981.

Vachon, Mary L. "Motivation and Stress Experienced by Staff Working with the Terminally Ill." *Death Education* 2 (1978): 117.

──────. "Staff Stress in Care of the Terminally Ill." In *Hospice Care: Principles and Practice.* ed. Charles Corr and Donna Corr. New York: Springer Publishing, 1983.

Weller, Stella. "Unending Thoughts." *Nursing Mirror* April 30, 1981, pp. 20-22.

White House Conference on Aging, 1981. *Executive Summary of Technical Committee on Creating an Age Integrated Society: Implications for Spiritual Well-Being.* Washington, D.C.: U.S. Government Printing Office, 1981.

Case Example

Home-Health-Agency-Based Hospice

Sylvia H. Schraff

Home care of the terminally ill is not a new idea to those who provide home health services in the community. Community health nurses have cared for the dying and their families ever since public health agencies and visiting nurse associations were established. Many of these organizations were hampered in their efforts to care for the dying by the restrictions imposed by third-party payors, whose reimbursement rules were based on the curative model of care.

When the hospice movement began to pick up momentum, however, members of the public started to recognize the special needs of the dying and the inappropriateness of the current system of care. Some of these newly informed people were volunteers who served on boards and advisory committees of human service organizations, some were professional health care providers, others were businesspersons, members of the clergy, and community leaders. These people began exploring the hospice concept and the feasibility of bringing such programs to their communities. Some of these people sought out their community health agencies to explore their ability to expand their roles. So it was with the Home Nursing Agency and how the agency came to develop a hospice program for the terminally ill in our area.

The Home Nursing Agency was established in 1968 by a group of community citizens who were interested in bringing needed home care services to the ill and disabled in their community. The agency began by providing services in Blair County and later expanded into the adjacent counties of Huntingdon, Fulton, and Bedford. Our service area, south-central Pennsylvania, is predominantly rural. A group of community-minded persons organized the agency as a voluntary nonprofit corporation, sought out community support and resources, established policy, and hired the staff to initiate services. The agency obtained certification as a Medicare provider of home health services and initially provided nursing, physical and speech therapy, and social work services on a visiting basis in the home.

Today the Home Nursing Agency is a multiprogram, multicounty organization serving a population base of approximately 230,000 with a staff of over 425 and an annual budget in excess of $5,000,000. In addition to the home health and hospice programs, the agency operates a community support program for the mentally ill that includes a licensed partial-hospitalization service as part of the overall mental health system; a maternal-child program that includes pre- and postnatal care, health teaching, and child care as well as a women's, infants', and children's supplemental feeding program (WIC); and a supportive care program through which homemaker and home health aide, chore, companion, respite, and private-duty services are available. The agency has evolved in response to the community's needs and concerns over the 15 years it has been in existence and has enjoyed a close working relationship with area physicians, hospitals, nursing homes, and other human service providers. The hospice program, which began in 1979, was an outgrowth of this responsiveness and close working relationship with allied health care providers.

HISTORICAL PERSPECTIVE

In reviewing the materials developed in planning and implementing the hospice program of the Home Nursing Agency, I was impressed with the sequence of events that led to the current program. When one is close to the day-to-day activities, one tends not to have a clear perspective of historical development but rather to be more concerned with solving current problems. The Home Nursing Agency's hospice program is a good example of a concept of care evolving into a formal program of service. I would like to describe this evolution and some of the significant events that led to the program as it exists today.

Identification of Need

The medical advisory committee to the Home Nursing Agency's board of directors undertook the effort to determine if a specialized care program for the terminally ill was needed. During 1977 and 1978, an analysis of the agency's caseload revealed that approximately 360 terminally ill persons had received home care. Discussions with staff members revealed the frustrations they felt in caring for these individuals: their lack of education in the care of the dying and the lack of a uniform model of care within the medical community. Physicians who referred patients often had difficulty accepting that their patients were terminally ill. Some physicians refused to tell patients that they were dying. Others referred patients to the agency but were reluctant to participate in the design of any plan of care that was noncurative in nature. Fortunately, there were some physicians who understood palliative care and who, together with the nursing staff, provided care that eased the suffering of the dying and helped them live their remaining days to the fullest. It was knowledge of these rewarding situations that prompted the medical advisory committee as well as staff members to examine the need for a specialized program of care.

It was recognized early that the community's acceptance of and cooperation with the program were essential to its success. The Home Nursing Agency was established by and for the communities it served and therefore felt it necessary to determine if there was support for a specialized program for the terminally ill as well as a perceived need for such a program. It was felt that advice and opinions should be sought from the medical community, allied human-services organizations, the Health Systems Agency, and the community at large, as represented by the agency's advisory professional committee.

The advisory committee is composed of physicians and allied health professionals from throughout the agency's service area. The committee members' informal discussions with their colleagues revealed agreement not only on the need for such a program but also that the Home Nursing Agency was the best location for it. Furthermore, a survey of patients' records showed that of the 190 physicians practicing in the area, 113 had referred people for terminal care. Hospitals, nursing homes, social service agencies, and organizations such as the Cancer Society were contacted and also gave their support and encouragement. All of these human-service organizations expressed a need for appropriate care for the dying, and most felt that the home was the most appropriate setting for care.

The Health Systems Plan of the Keystone Health Systems Agency was reviewed and found to contain a specific objective regarding hospice services in the six-county area: "By 1983, support services of visiting professionals, including doctors, nurses, therapists and counselors, will be available to the terminally ill choosing to die at home" (p. 4). The plan also included the following recommended action: "Establish county-wide support organizations to encourage development of hospice services throughout the region. These organizations will also provide educational services on the hospice concept to both consumers and providers in the region" (p. 5). The Specialized Care Task Force of the Keystone Health Systems Agency initially developed the objective and recommendation in order to encourage the use of home-care hospice services. It was further felt by the task force that hospice services could be implemented sooner and more economically through a home care program. The Keystone Health Systems Agency later formalized its support for this endeavor in a letter accompanying the agency's request to participate in the Western Pennsylvania Blue Cross demonstration program for hospice care.

The advisory professional committee of the Home Nursing Agency's board of directors is composed of representatives of professional disciplines of service provided by the agency as well as laypersons interested in and knowledgeable about the human-service sector of their community. This committee has the responsibility for recommending to the board all policy for service provision as well as ensuring quality care through research, evaluation, record review, and audit. This committee was also requested to review the need for and feasibility of establishing a special program for the terminally ill, and late in 1978 it recommended that the board of directors establish a hospice program. The board received a similar recommendation from the medical advisory committee, and at its annual meeting in January 1979 directed the staff to proceed with the project.

Program Development

In accordance with the official directive of the board, the staff set about developing the program and preparing grant proposals to secure financial assistance. Of utmost importance was the need to respond to the Health Care Financing Administration's request for proposals, published in the *Federal Register* of October 27, 1978. Proposals were being sought from organizations willing to participate in a national demonstration project. Therefore, the data we had collected were amassed and our plans for development of the hospice were outlined. In addition, a proposal was prepared in the spring of 1979 for a demonstration of the cost effectiveness of hospice care to be conducted by Blue Cross of Western Pennsylvania.

In the meantime, the agency staff began to formulate plans for the development of the hospice. From the beginning, we decided to utilize the concept of a hospice home-care team, to be composed of nurses, aides, therapists, and social workers specially trained to provide care to the dying. The agency at that time utilized a team approach to the delivery of home care services. Teams were either geographic in focus or specialized, such as the team for maternal-child services. Since the concept of specialized care teams was already familiar to the agency, it would be relatively simple to utilize this concept to begin building the program.

Since the agency was certified as a home health agency under the special provision of Title 18 of the Social Security Act and had been providing skilled nursing and therapeutic service to persons dying at home, funding the special hospice team was not considered to be a problem as long as services were limited to those covered under the regulations. Also, the agency had an active volunteer program, providing volunteer services to homebound patients.

A survey of the records of terminally ill patients served during the previous two years showed that of approximately 360 patients, 61 percent were Medicare patients, 14 percent were Medicaid patients, 15 percent were covered by private insurance, and 10 percent paid for services directly. Since the agency received money from the United Way, the county government, and local municipalities and townships to subsidize care for persons without adequate insurance coverage or means to afford the full cost of care, the financial risk of caring for the relatively low number of partial-fee patients was felt to be minimal, at least for a beginning program.

Development of a philosophy of care, program goals, policies, and training courses were the next activities undertaken. In order to ensure that the program developed in accord with the national hospice movement, it was felt best to familiarize a staff member with a recognized program. The agency's assistant director attended a workshop conducted by the Yale-New Haven Hospice in the spring of 1979.

At this stage of program development, the hospice philosophy of care was explored as well as the goals to be achieved. It was decided at this time to limit the program to a specialized team that would provide care designed to help terminally ill patients and their families cope with the reality of the terminal illness and live their remaining days of life as comfortably as possible. Palliative care measures were researched and identified for use in the program. Patients would be admitted to the program in accord with their needs and the capabilities of staff. Patients who had not been informed of their terminal state would be accepted as well as those who had.

A definition and statement of purpose were developed by the advisory professional committee and staff members. The hospice home care team was defined as "a caring community dedicated to providing comfort and care to clients and families who are dealing with an incurable illness with a limited prognosis (weeks or months)." The hospice home care team was seen to function in the hope that the client and family might be able to prepare for death in a way that is satisfactory to them. The components of the program were as follows:

1. Physician-directed service.//
2. Care by a multidisciplinary team.
3. Access to all home-care services: nursing, therapy, social service, homemaker/home health aide service.
4. 24-hour service.
5. Client and family regarded as the unit of care.
6. Special attention to control of symptoms.
7. Volunteer program.
8. Bereavement follow-up.

The policies of the existing home-care program were used to guide the staff in providing care. It soon became apparent that there was a need for specific procedures for pain control and symptom relief, and the staff subsequently developed these. New policies for personnel in the specialized team were approved by the board of directors in the fall of 1979 to allow for additional time off and reimbursement for on-call hours.

Volunteers were seen as an essential component of the home-care team. The agency staff members were experienced in using volunteers to supplement the home care program, since the agency sponsored a large Retired Senior Volunteer Program (RSVP). RSVP volunteers were selected for their interest and experience and were given training and orientation in the special needs of the dying.

Bereavement visits were early recognized as important in the after-care of surviving family members. Initially, the nurses on the hospice home care team performed this service through home visits or follow-up phone calls. Later, volunteers provided this care.

Agency staff members were selected to receive the initial three-week training course. Not all staff members who participated in the course were selected for the initial team, nor were staff members obligated to continue the program if they became uncomfortable with the idea of hospice care. From the initial group, three nurses, two aides, and a social worker were selected for the hospice home care team. In addition to the training of staff, the agency provided in-service education programs to local hospitals, physicians, and nurses in order to acquaint them with the concept of hospice and methods of referral. Such public-relations efforts proved so successful that one week before the program officially opened, the agency received seven referrals specifically for hospice care. The new service began on September 1, 1979.

Evolution of the Program

With the hospice home care team established, the agency began to explore ways to educate the community as well as introduce the program to all service areas. Although the agency was not chosen as one of the hospice programs to receive funding under the national demonstration project, the decision was made to proceed with plans as originally formulated. Training programs were conducted for selected staff members in all geographic service areas, and teams of specialists were identified in accord with caseload. Slide programs were developed to assist the agency in educating the community. Interest in the program was high, and staff members were frequently called upon to tell the special story of hospice.

The newly developed team met on a daily basis and worked closely together in designing plans of care for their patients. Referrals came from physicians, hospitals, and the community at large as well as from home care staff within the agency. Such transfers from co-workers were often delayed or difficult to achieve, as staff members often became attached to their patients and were reluctant to turn them over to another team. Hospice home care staff frequently had to convince their co-workers to transfer their terminally ill patients early enough so that their special skills could best be put to use.

Issues and Conflicts. The issue of a generalist versus a specialist approach to providing care soon emerged among the staff. Home care staff resented the special treatment, such as additional time off, that was given to hospice team members, as well as all the attention they received. Staff members who had been caring for terminally ill patients for years questioned the need for a specialized care team. They requested special inservice education programs and training on the care of the dying, which they felt would be relevant to the care of other patients.

In the meantime, the hospice home care team soon began to feel the effects of 24-hour availability of service. Nurses who were on call for a week at a time needed extra days off to recover from the stress and anxiety of such demands. It was decided to solve this problem by giving all staff members the opportunity to participate in the hospice training program, after which hospice clients could be absorbed into the overall agency on-call system. This new system alleviated the need for two agency nurses to be on call and had the subsequent effect of reducing each agency nurse's on-call period to a frequency of less than twice a year. Correspondingly, hospice home care staff members' anxiety and stress were reduced, and additional time off was no longer needed.

As the program evolved, additional fallout from the effort to train all staff members soon became apparent. Instead of transferring their patients earlier, home care staff, armed with their new knowledge, became even more reluctant to transfer their patients to the hospice team. It was decided to allow selected patients to receive care from members of the home care staff, provided that the home care staff presented the case to the hospice team, worked with the team in designing the plan of care, and coordinated all care with the team leader. This worked for a time, but the agency was experiencing other changes that soon had a profound effect on the new program.

During 1981, the agency began to move to a primary nursing model rather than continue with the team approach. Primary nursing was felt to hold many advantages for both the patient and the caregiver. Home care patients would have a specific nurse who was responsible for providing care or facilitating the provision of care. Primary-care nurses would be assigned geographic districts and would have associate and assisting nurses to help them provide for their patients. Hospice nurses would be primary nurses for their geographic areas and coordination of care would be accomplished through weekly case conferences. Home care staff members could provide care to hospice patients as long as they utilized case conferences to coordinate care and elicited input for care planning.

Soon it became evident that the program was losing its identity. Nurses who were caring for patients within the curative or rehabilitation models had difficulty switching to a palliative care approach for a few of their patients. Bereavement follow-up was inconsistent, as was the use of volunteers. The medical community likewise had not progressed in their understanding of and use of palliative care.

As with any home health program, inpatient care was provided at the physician's discretion and coordination of care from inpatient institution to home was carried out by the institution's social service department and the agency's liaison nurse. Hospitals and nursing homes were most cooperative in their efforts to ensure a continuity of care, but problems still arose. Notable were the problems that occurred when patients were transferred from the home care program to hospitals. If the patient was admitted to the hospital when his primary physician was away, delays in ordering pain-control medications resulted, thus increasing the patient's suffering. Some hospitals permitted hospice personnel and volunteers to visit at any time and welcomed the coordination of care plans. Others restricted such visiting and were not receptive to joint planning. Hospice staff members used ingenious methods to continue to work with their patients and were frequently successful in thwarting what might have been difficult experiences for their patients.

Reorganization

Fortunately, hospice providers moved to bring about legislation to support hospices and set some standard for the industry. There was an evident need to reestablish the team approach for hospice, get on with the task of educating the health care community, and establish cooperative agreements with hospitals and nursing homes for inpatient care. In March 1982, the agency's medical advisory committee, after studying the results of audits and reports from staff, recommended that the board of directors establish a full hospice program, as opposed to the more limited hospice home care team. The agency staff was directed to investigate the feasibility of hiring a medical director, establishing an interdisciplinary team, and arranging for coordination of inpatient care. The planning committee of the board of directors and the advisory professional committee concurred with the recommendation of the medical advisory committee and called for the development of a separate statement of philosophy and goals as well as distinct policies and procedures that would set the program apart from home care. And so in April 1982, the agency redirected its efforts in hospice.

The first step was to appoint a hospice director and to choose the members of the team. A nurse-director was appointed and nurses in each geographic area were selected to provide hospice service. Social workers and therapists in all geographic areas were likewise selected and trained to participate in the care of the terminally ill as needed. Later, as the program evolved, a director of volunteers was selected as well as a spiritual counselor. The medical director was appointed in April 1983.

The need for hospice care was reaffirmed within the agency. The team of hospice workers and volunteers reaffirmed the special nature of hospice care, and the agency's staff were soon convinced that the team did indeed have unique capabilities. The number of referrals was overwhelming: over 300 persons received hospice care in 1982.

In addition to separating out hospice as a cost center, the agency had to separate the hospice program from the home health program. Statements of philosophy and goals as well as policies and procedures were developed by a hospice subcommittee of the advisory professional committee. The medical director and medical advisory committee began developing protocols to be used for hospice patients. Educational efforts were also undertaken with the health care community.

Medicare Certification. In the midst of this growth, the national legislation on hospice was approved in November 1982 to become effective the following November. The committees of the board recommended that the agency be certified as a hospice under Medicare, and the board authorized the staff to begin the process. One of the initial steps was to address the need to coordinate inpatient service.

The board took the position that hospice patients should have inpatient services available to them as close to their homes as possible in institutions used by their own physicians. In the four-county area, there were 8 hospitals and 11 nursing homes. Some of the hospitals expressed interest in creating special hospice units, and the feasibility of such endeavors was explored. At one hospital a pilot project was instituted to ascertain the need for such a unit. Generally, the feeling in the hospitals was that because of the limitations of the new legislation and the emphasis on home care, the expense of creating special hospice units could not be justified.

The agency drafted agreements and held meetings with hospital and nursing home administrators. Concern was expressed about the low rate of Medicare reimbursement as well as the risks that would be taken by both the agency and the inservice institutions. Administrators wanted clarification of the role of the medical director and the authority of the attending physician. Discussions were held on the mechanics of coordinating care, the role of the hospice team, and inpatient visiting privileges for hospice staff. For the most part, hospitals and nursing homes were supportive as well as encouraging. Nursing homes that chose not to participate did so only because of their lack of flexibility in assigning available beds. At the time of the agency's site visit for certification, two large hospitals and one nursing home had agreed to participate in the program, and their staffs subsequently received special training. Other hospitals and nursing homes agreed to participate later.

An agreement for drugs and biologicals was drafted and sent to local pharmacies. In order to participate, local pharmacies had to agree to make certain commonly used medications available on a 24-hour basis, accept the average wholesale price (AWP) plus a small dispensing fee, and accept return of unused controlled narcotics and destroy them in accordance with regulations. The response was greater than anticipated and agreements were secured throughout the four-county area.

December 1983 was the date of our site visit for certification of the hospice program. The representative from the Pennsylvania State Health Department pored over our records, interviewed staff members and volunteers, attended case conferences, and scrutinized policies and coordination agreements. In February 1984, the agency was officially notified that it was certified retroactively to December 21, 1983, as a hospice, the first visiting nurse agency in Pennsylvania to be so certified.

THE CURRENT PROGRAM

The Home Nursing Agency's hospice program developed steadily throughout the five years of its existence. Today the program has a staff of 13 and an active daily caseload of approximately 40 patients throughout the geographic areas of service. At this writing the program has been Medicare certified for approximately eight months and therefore has some experience in working with this new benefit.

Coordination of Care

Coordination of care is one difficulty encountered in serving a large multicounty area. The agency has six offices located throughout the area, each with its own staff and supervisor. Hospice staff are designated in the outlying areas to provide care as part of the overall home health team. The agency has one designated interdisciplinary hospice team, located in the main office, that meets weekly to discuss admissions, plan patient care, and develop policies and procedures for the program. Hospice team members from the outlying geographic areas come to the weekly meetings to present their cases for admission as well as to elicit the help of the group in planning for care. Since some of the counties have rather small populations and anticipated yearly caseloads of fewer than 25 patients, this system will probably suffice for some time. However, it is becoming apparent that one of the larger counties will need its own interdisciplinary hospice team to assist more directly with day-to-day care planning. Policy development would still remain with the team in the main office. This situation is being studied at the present time for its impact on quality of care as well as efficiency.

Financing

The hospice program uses the new Medicare hospice benefit as well as the traditional home health benefits available through Medicare, Medicaid, and other third-party payors. The agency also has contracts for homemaker service under the Title 20 and area Agency on Aging programs and supplements the care of families as needed with this service. The interdisciplinary team recommends the funding source under which a patient is to be admitted and determines level of service in accordance with the patient's needs and the eligibility standards.

Early in the program, the agency decided that its hospice program should serve all persons in need and be flexible enough to accommodate the special eligibility and service requirements imposed by various funding agencies. As a result, the agency's generic policies for hospice can accommodate persons who wish to opt for the new Medicare program, those who elect not to participate, as well as anyone else who has the need for hospice care, regardless of age or payment source. This position has proved to be beneficial for all concerned. Today the majority of patients are still being cared for under the home health benefit. As experience is gained and staff members become more secure in their own capabilities, the new Medicare benefit will most likely gain in popularity.

Current Program Parameters

Current statistics show that approximately 20 percent of all hospice patients are below the age of 60; data on length of stay show that 79 percent of all patients die within three months of admission. Hospitals account for the majority of referrals, with family or self referrals ranking second. Physicians refer approximately 15 percent of all patients. The caseload has varied throughout the years: 1982 showed a high of 303 persons served, while 167 were served in 1983. The current year (1984) is expected to equal 1982, especially in the new climate of prospective payment (DRGs) for hospital care. An average of 13 nursing visits are made for each hospice patient, while home-health-aide visits average 18 and social service visits average 2 per patient. The hospice counselor sees approximately 16 percent of all clients, as requested by the team. Volunteer hours have totaled 2,159 in the past year. An average of 53 percent of patients opt to have the support of volunteers.

Staffing changes have also occurred over the years. New staff members have been added to the team to fill new as well as vacated positions. The nurse-director moved on and was replaced by a director who was a social worker by profession. A clinical nurse specialist was then hired as the nursing supervisor. Other staff members, such as the counselor, medical director, volunteer director, and home health aides, have remained with the program. Recently the position of program director became vacant again and a new director had to be hired. In spite of such fluctuation, the staff have remained a stable and cohesive group. They are dedicated to their program and work enthusiastically to make their services available to those in need.

The medical director of the program has established a good working relationship with area physicians. He has been instrumental in helping them understand the concept of palliative care and frequently serves as a liaison between the primary physician and the hospice staff. In addition, he and the clinical nurse specialist continue to develop procedures and protocols for patient care.

Volunteers have proven to be one of the greatest assets to the program. It is extremely rewarding to all involved to see the personal dedication and spirit of caring possessed by these people. The director of volunteers trained a group of 24 to serve the main office and later trained volunteers in the outlying counties.

These people work tirelessly and willingly do whatever is needed. Their dedication and support has made the difference in many instances in helping families keep their promise to allow their loved one to die at home. Today the volunteers do most of the bereavement visits and have formed a special bereavement support group to assist each other in their mission. Many additional activities are being planned to help utilize the many talents of these dedicated people.

ISSUES AND CONSIDERATIONS

As I look back over the past years and see the difference in our level of awareness about the special needs of the dying, I am most impressed by as well as grateful to those who instituted the hospice movement. People across the nation are aware of hospice and support the concept and the emphasis on keeping people as comfortable as possible in the environment of their choice. The medical and nursing communities are feeling the rewards of delivering palliative care. But most of all, people are coming to grips with the knowledge that dying is a part of living and that death can be accomplished in a healthy fashion.

Yet there is still much to be done. Education is still a major goal—education not only of the health care community but also of the general population. We must break the habit of shielding ourselves and our loved ones from the pain of death, adopt a more healthy attitude, and accept our mortality.

As I look over the program and think of tomorrow, I know that we still need to educate health care professionals to refer patients to hospice earlier, while there is still time to help them. Physicians as well as nurses are reluctant to give up. Even now, home care staff members occasionally refer a patient for hospice care when life expectancy is only a few days. We must find ways to prevent these problems and recognize the health care professional's difficulty in dealing with death.

Financing of hospice services continues to be a concern. If our agency had to depend only on the new Medicare legislation for hospice care, we would have given up by now. The home health benefit provided by third-party payors continues to be our major resource. Community funds, as well as gifts and contributions, are used to subsidize the care of patients who do not have adequate resources or insurance. As demands for home care continue to grow, I worry that the limited community dollars available will be stretched beyond their ability to provide care to all in need.

Another problem that I can see developing in some areas is competition with other hospices and home health organizations. Some people say that competition is healthy, while others feel that it results in higher costs and lower quality of care. Each side has a point, but it is nevertheless an issue that must be studied.

The last concern I have is for the concept of two distinct modes of care: palliative and curative. Is it realistic to believe that each model is all encompassing? Must a patient or caregiver choose one model over the other? Must one model be exclusive of the other? These questions have been raised by our staff ever since the hospice program began. Our dilemma was implied in my statement that we accept some patients who have not been told of their terminal illness. Obviously, some of our hospice patients who receive care under their home health benefit are receiving care that is classified as curative. The hospice staff feels that hospice care can be beneficial regardless of the model of care or treatment regimen. Is the issue palliative versus curative care, or is it healthy dying regardless of the route followed?

FUTURE PLANS

The goal that continues to guide the growth and direction of the hospice program is that which was formulated at the inception of the program: to develop a caring community dedicated to providing comfort and care to patients and their families who are dealing with an incurable illness with a limited prognosis. This statement has many implications.

Development of a caring community includes more than the caring of the interdisciplinary team. Our goal statement focuses on the community as a whole, including the human service sector, the political community, religious groups, volunteer organizations, as well as the community at large.

Of special importance is the need to develop networks of support groups working together to help the patient and family. Special-interest groups within churches seem to hold a great potential for bringing talent and expertise to the program. Establishing such linkages and developing means of coordinating the work they do is one of our future goals.

Reaching out to physicians and eliciting their support and cooperation will continue to be a major endeavor. Looking at innovative ways to help each other, to share our respective expertise, and to encourage the timely use of our hospice service will be an ongoing effort. Education is not the sole answer. Innovative ways must be developed to break through the barrier of avoidance of death. Trusting relationships must be formed and a partnership approach adopted if we are to reach all those in need.

Our staff is currently developing protocols that give them alternative strategies to use in pain control and comfort measures. Physicians will have the option to choose to use these measures as the need arises. Development of such standards and allowing for choice should be a step toward encouraging a trusting, collegial relationship.

Finally, community support must be continually cultivated and encouraged, support not only in the sense of monetary gifts but also in the sense of guidance, time, talent, and understanding. The community will continue to be the agency's reason for being and the focus of its activities, now and in the future.

SUMMARY

The Home Nursing Agency's hospice program evolved from the dreams and the hopes of many people. The movement from an idea to a reality takes many steps and many changes in people's ways of thinking, understanding, and acting. I have tried to depict the process whereby a home health agency's program of caring for the ill and disabled in their own environment expanded into a special service for the terminally ill. Through this sharing of our experience, I hope others may gain insight and the knowledge required to realize their own dreams about hospice.

Case Example

A Community Based Hospice

Myra J. Downs

The need for a community-wide hospice program for Etowah County, Alabama, was formally documented by community health nursing students in November 1983; however, many informal discussions among various groups had been taking place for years. In order to meet their requirements for an educational project, three senior nursing students planned and implemented a seminar entitled "Hospice: A Community Need?" They brought speakers from the nearby Birmingham Area Hospice to discuss and explain the hospice concept to the local community as well as to describe their experiences with hospice care. In addition, a local minister whose background included serving as a hospital chaplain and a home missionary was included in the program to help identify where hospice services could be of benefit in the local area. Overall, the seminar was very successful. More than 150 local citizens attended the well-publicized seminar, and approximately 60 people volunteered their services to help organize or work in a hospice program.

Etowah County is a rural area in northwest Alabama. The largest town is Gadsden, a city of approximately 50,000 people. The county is in the area known as the Bible Belt, and approximately 60 percent of the population declare themselves to be Southern Baptists. Therefore it seemed appropriate for the Etowah Baptist Association (EBA) and Baptist Health Services, Inc. (BHS), to be involved in the formation of the hospice program.

Among those in attendance at the community-wide seminar were officials from EBA and BHS. EBA is a county organization that works with the more than 80 Baptist churches in the community, and BHS is a corporation that owns the larger of the two hospitals in the community as well as other health care facilities. Representatives from each of these groups began talking after the seminar and felt that they should respond to the needs of the community. Because I had experience in hospice program organization, I was contacted to serve as a consultant. Thus the ball began to roll.

TYPE OF PROGRAM NEEDED

It was determined early in the planning stages that the community needed a hospice program that would provide care to all people in the community without regard to religious preference, race, sex, or economic status. The officials from both Baptist organizations wanted the entire community to benefit from the program, not just those of the Baptist faith. A staff person from EBA and one from BHS were appointed to join me in a task force to plan and implement the program. This small group developed the organizational plan to identify the resources needed for the hospice program.

COMMUNITY-WIDE ADVISORY BOARD

The first order of business was to appoint an advisory board, made up of representatives of various disciplines and lay persons, that could represent the entire community. A list of approximately 20 names was put together, and the task force members contacted each person, either by phone or in person, to find out if he or she wished to serve on the advisory board. Many of those contacted had previously expressed an interest in hospice either through informal discussions or attendance at the hospice seminar. Others were contacted because of their position in the community or their history of leadership. Because public relations and community education are important, especially early in program development, a person with a background in public relations was included. The only oncologist in the area was also invited to participate. Overall, the people chosen were those who could bring specific strengths to the new program.

The advisory group held its first meeting in February 1984, at which time the task force presented a program on the hospice concept and set out a tentative plan for the future local program. Specific goals were identified and many members of the advisory group offered assistance.

A statement of philosophy for the program was an essential first step. The board reviewed and adopted the hospice philosophy developed by the National Hospice Organization:

> Hospice affirms life. Hospice exists to provide support and care for persons in the last phases of incurable disease so that they may live as fully and comfortably as possible. Hospice services are available on the basis of need and not on the basis of ability to pay. Hospice is available to persons without regard to race, creed, color or national origin. Hospice recognizes dying as a normal process whether or not resulting from disease. Hospice neither hastens nor postpones death. Hospice exists in the hope and belief that, through appropriate care and the promotion of a caring community sensitive to their needs, patients and families may be free to attain a degree of mental and philosophical preparation for death that is satisfactory to them.

The philosophy provided a base on which to build the program.

Various details were also addressed at this time, such as designation of a recording secretary to keep minutes of the meetings, time and place for future meetings, others in the community who could serve on the advisory board. The overall interest and enthusiasm of the board members was strong, which was additional evidence of the community's need for the program.

ORGANIZATION AND ADMINISTRATION

Since BHS had experience in health care, it was decided that they could lend technical assistance in the area of administration. The staff person from BHS therefore began negotiating with the various health facilities to supply needed resources, such as a nurse coordinator, office space and telephone, supplies, and so forth. The Baptist Hospital agreed to supply a nurse part-time to provide nursing leadership and coordination. The Professional Office Building (POB) found office space and a phone, and a foundation office set up a special fund to accept tax-deductible donations.

The advisory board also worked closely with BHS. Officers (president, vice-president, secretary, and financial chairman) were elected. Committees on professional standards, volunteer activities, public relations, and fund raising were set up to assist with the development of the hospice program administration and organization.

Recruitment and Training of Volunteers

The EBA staff person took the responsibility of working with the chairman of the volunteer activities committee. Since the EBA worked with approximately 80 different churches in the area and had lists of many members who already volunteered their time, it was thought that they could recruit some of the volunteers needed to work in the program. It was also determined that through community awareness, created by newspaper articles, notices in church bulletins, and so forth, other volunteers could be recruited.

The EBA staff member, the advisory board volunteer activities committee, and I worked closely together to plan the volunteer training program. It was determined that two 3-hour sessions would serve as the initial training, with monthly inservice programs to follow. Also, the volunteer applicants would have to have a personal interview with a screening committee before being accepted in the program. When the volunteers accumulated 12 hours of training, they would receive a certificate documenting their involvement and education.

The agenda for the first training session included an overview of hospice, presented by the nurse coordinator of a hospice program from another part of the state; spiritual issues, discussed by a panel of ministers; death and dying issues, as perceived by a physician; as well as the plans for the local hospice program. Another important aspect of the training program included the role of the volunteer, both professional and lay, in the hospice program.

The sessions were held on consecutive Tuesday and Thursday evenings at the public library, a place that was considered to be inviting to potential volunteers from many different areas and of all faiths. Approximately 60 volunteers attended the training sessions and decided on the area in which they wanted to volunteer: direct patient care, bereavement, public relations, or clerical. Small-group work was also a part of the sessions, which allowed the interest groups time to get to know each other and make plans.

Professional Volunteers

The nurse-coordinator and I also recruited and trained registered nurse volunteers for the program. The volunteers came from various areas of nursing, such as anesthesia, nursing homes, intensive care, and home health; therefore, continuing education in the area of hospice nursing care was essential. It was determined that in addition to specific programs on such topics as pain and symptom control, the weekly team meeting would serve as an arena for learning.

Recruitment for membership on the interdisciplinary team did not prove to be difficult. Because the hospice program was a total community effort, members of various disciplines from throughout the area were eager to participate. Several people, when contacted, told us that they had worked with hospice programs in other areas and could bring experience to the team. Scheduling a meeting time convenient to all team members proved somewhat of a problem; however, the medical director and other team members were so anxious to get started that weekly brown-bag lunchtime team meetings were established, with the Baptist Hospital donating classroom space. A suggested team format for coordinating each patient's care was adopted, and the team, made up of a mixture of people from throughout the community, was ready to serve.

Policies and Procedures

Another major step was the development of appropriate policies and procedures. Job descriptions for each member of the team were developed, using models from other hospice programs (see Chapter 4) modified to make them specific to the local program. At the first team meeting, the draft job descriptions were given to each team member for their opinions. The professional standards committee of the advisory board also reviewed the job descriptions. After both groups had made recommendations, the job descriptions were finalized and presented to the full advisory board for approval, with the recommendation that the team review them six months after implementation of the program, since it was believed that using the documents was the best way to test their completeness and validity.

Writing protocols for such items as program admission and the geographic area of program coverage, as well as program policies and procedures, was a joint effort of the professional team and the advisory board. Because the nurse-coordinator and medical director attended the monthly advisory board meetings, communication was very good and decisions could be made that were both practical and effective for the overall program.

The board also had to develop bylaws for the organization. A local attorney volunteered his time and resources to the board, and within a short period of time a legal structure was set up that had appropriate authority to conduct the business of the program.

Team Support

A local psychologist voiced interest in working in the hospice program early in the planning stages. It was decided that in such a small community-wide program he would need to wear several hats. He agreed to serve as a consultant to the team members, especially in the area of therapeutic communication; provide direct services (without a fee) to patients or their families; and lead the hospice team support group. Because the team members would be coming to the weekly team meetings from various areas of the community, it was decided to hold support group meetings immediately after the team meeting, either on a monthly basis or as needed. This particular arrangement has worked well during the early months of program implementation, but as the program continues to grow the frequency of the support group meetings may need to be changed.

FINANCIAL STRUCTURE

Etowah County Hospice Organization (ECHO) is a not-for-profit structure relying on donations and grants for its existence. The Baptist Hospital funded a half-time nurse position (.5 FTE) for the nurse-coordinator for the program as well as donating space in the POB for an office. The Baptist Health Services Corporation provided seed money for such items as equipment, stationery, and educational expenses. Several other businesses and agencies have donated items to the program. Other funding sources, such as the United Way and the local Cancer Society, have voiced an interest in the program. Proposals are being written in order to secure these funds.

The agency also plans to meet the standards and file application for Medicare reimbursement. The BHS will provide the administrative assistance necessary to reach this goal.

The financial support of the agency is increasing. There is committed support in the local community, and fund-raising events are being planned by volunteers.

BEREAVEMENT PROGRAM

Although there are several schools of thought regarding who should handle bereavement, it has been the experience of this hospice program that the volunteers who work with the family before the patient's death can be effective in working with the survivors. In one particular situation, a retarded daughter of the hospice patient formed a friendship with a volunteer who was working with the family. The volunteer felt that it would be devastating to the daughter to experience the loss of her friend in addition to the loss of her mother. Therefore, the volunteer worked with the daughter and other family members during the bereavement period. This proved to be a good experience for all involved.

The nurse-coordinator and the psychologist work closely with the volunteers during the bereavement period. The volunteers need support both to work through their own grief and help the family regain the independence they might have lost.

The bereavement program is modeled after many others in that significant dates, such as birthdays and anniversaries, are kept in a tickler file and relatives of the patient are contacted on the days. Because grief is as individual as the person experiencing it, the volunteers attempt to identify the particular needs of each survivor and work to meet these needs.

QUALITY ASSURANCE

Quality assurance is an important aspect of any health care program, and hospice is no exception. There are several components of the ECHO quality assurance program. One is peer review. The nurse-coordinator visits each hospice family on admission and at least once each month in order to assist the primary nurse in planning the care of the patient and family. In addition, the team meeting, which allows for peer review by the interdisciplinary team, serves as a portion of the overall quality assurance program.

Another component of the program is the quality care committee, which is composed of four professionals from the community and meets quarterly to review active patient records and make recommendations regarding the care being provided. A report is given to the nurse-coordinator and the professional standards committee of the advisory board.

In addition questionnaires about level of satisfaction with the program are mailed to all patients and their physicians. The quality care committee reviews the responses to these questionnaires on a quarterly basis and makes a report to both the hospice nurse-coordinator and the professional standards committee of the advisory board.

Volunteers are involved in the quality assurance program in that the volunteer chairman visits with each volunteer initially and periodically throughout the service period. The coordinator also attends team meetings and talks with each volunteer frequently about the family's needs, responses, and so forth. Many patients have two volunteers working in the home. This allows for informal peer review but mainly serves as a means of peer support as well as providing dependability and continuity of care for the family.

EPILOGUE

The seed of ECHO was planted in November 1983 at a community-wide seminar. The next six months were a time for planning, securing resources, training caregivers, and providing further community education. The interdisciplinary team began serving patients in June 1984. Because of careful planning and tremendous community involvement, the program is being widely accepted and used. One area that caused some concern and required a policy change was patient referral to the program. Initially, our policy stated the nurse-coordinator would make one assessment visit on the recommendation of the hospital discharge planner or a family request. She would then consult with the patient's physician to obtain his specific orders for care. One physician felt that this was taking away his control of his patient. Although the nurses in the program disagreed with his argument, it was determined that since the program was in its infancy it was best not to alienate any member of the medical staff, and therefore, for the good of the program, a policy change was made to incorporate discussion with the primary physician before the assessment visit.

Overall, whether in a small hospice such as this one or a larger program, good, effective communication appears to be the ingredient necessary for the success of the program. Incorporating fluid channels of communication among all parties will definitely decrease problems and enhance success.

Case Example

Merger of Hospice and VNA

S. Jill Schultz

BACKGROUND

Saginaw, Michigan, is a mid-sized community with a population of more than 200,000 people. Its largest employer is the General Motors Corporation. The existing health care system consists of four acute-care hospitals, a Veteran's Administration hospital, a rehabilitation hospital, approximately 300 physicians, a Visiting Nurse Association (VNA), the county health department, a proprietary home health agency, and an assortment of related service organizations.

In 1976-77 a group of concerned health professionals established a support group to help cancer patients and their families cope with cancer. In addition to providing support, the group identified the needs to approach the terminally ill and their families in a more humane fashion and to educate the community about the needs of the terminally ill. The original group consisted of spiritual leaders, cancer victims and their families, a physician, nurses from various institutions and agencies, social workers, and health care administrators.

At the time, the hospice concept was new, and hospice programs were beginning in other parts of the country. Several members of the group reviewed a hospice program that was established in a neighboring state and explored the literature on hospice, and on January 26, 1979, the group filed for incorporation with the state as the Hospice of Saginaw, Inc. (HOS). The purpose of the organization was "to help meet the physical, intellectual, emotional, and spiritual needs of terminally ill persons and their families and to educate the community of Saginaw and surrounding county about the needs of terminally ill persons and their families."

In February 1979 the Articles of Incorporation were approved as filed with the state of Michigan. Shortly thereafter, one of the original incorporators withdrew from the board and began developing a hospital-based hospice program.

The next year of hospice activities were primarily educational. Volunteer training and community education were provided by board members, who included representation from the VNA of Saginaw, and other volunteers. The decision to provide direct services was made in late 1979. Office space and services were financed through fund raising, and volunteers were used extensively.

In February 1980 the board of directors hired an executive director. Within several months a secretary was hired and Hospice of Saginaw was granted a 501c(3) tax-exempt status. A bank provided a grant of $20,000 to the new program.

Blue Cross/Blue Shield of Michigan had been in touch with Hospice of Saginaw to explore providing funding for the program through its Pilot Programs Division. It was at this point that the educational emphasis was shifted to actual provision of services.

Initially nursing services were provided by volunteers or through coordination with existing agencies' services. The VNA of Saginaw provided most of the nursing care and continued on the hospice board. In March 1981, Blue Cross/Blue Shield of Michigan initiated funding for Hospice of Saginaw, Inc. The amount of funding was to be based on the proportion of Blue Cross/Blue Shield clients served. The projection of the budget, including provisions for hiring more staff members, indicated that 50-60 percent of the budget would be funded through the grant. Application for funding through a local trust was also filed.

The political climate was crucial in the evolution of the program. The other, hospital-based, hospice program was viewed as unnecessary and duplicative. There was confusion among clients about which program they were involved with and who started first. Concurrently, there began a proliferation of home health care services in the community. One of the parties interested in providing home health services was the hospital that was developing a hospital-based hospice and opposition to the creation of additional programs increased the animosity between the hospice programs and existing home care agencies.

STEPS TO MERGER

In the late fall of 1981 the relationships between the VNA of Saginaw and HOS began to decline. While HOS opposed the hospital-based hospice and the hospital home care program, it began to explore the process of certification for home-health-agency status itself. This was opposed by the VNA. Hospice of Saginaw filed an application to become a certified home health agency in in January 1982. Patient services were provided by hospice staff members. Prior to the Michigan Department of Public Health survey for certification, internal difficulties developed. There was conflict between volunteers and agency administration. The medical directors resigned, and press coverage of the conflict damaged the program's credibility. Resolution occurred with the resignation of the executive director and patient care coordinator.

With the change in administration, there was a new director and a renewed effort to evaluate the direction the hospice program would take in the community. The program overcame the results of its unfavorable media coverage and continued providing services. The board of directors decided to withdraw the application for home health certification and explore alternatives that would allow the organization to remain viable.

In November 1982, the president of HOS met with the executive committee of the VNA because HOS was seeking to explore with the VNA the possibility of affiliation between the two agencies. The VNA established an ad hoc committee to review the feasibility of affiliation. The VNA board of directors recommended that the local United Way send a representative to the initial meeting between hospice and VNA representatives. The role of United Way was that of an interested party, since the VNA was an agency affiliate of United Way of Saginaw County and the Hospice of Saginaw had applied for admission to United Way in the past.

The ad hoc VNA committee analyzed the impact of affiliation with the hospice and concluded that there was potential value to the VNA. However, at the first meeting between representatives of both agencies, many questions were raised about legal and financial issues and management of services. To help find answers, the HOS board authorized the sharing of information between executive directors.

The results of meetings between the two directors were reported to both boards. Both directors felt that affiliation was possible from an operational standpoint. The two executive directors had the common goal of acting in the best interests of both organizations, regardless of personal interest. Had opposition or animosity developed at this time, the resulting merger would not have taken place.

The meeting of the representatives of both boards and of United Way led to a directive to hire an attorney to review legal means of meeting both agencies' needs. United Way's position was that agencies providing similar services should cooperate.

In the preliminary discussions, both agencies stated what they hoped to gain by affiliation. what areas could not be compromised, and which legal structure could best meet their needs.

The pros and cons of full corporate merger, parent-subsidiary relationship, and contractual affiliation were reviewed by both parties. After discussion, the HOS board representative determined that the hospice wanted to retain its name and logo and participate in decision making that concerned its services. The VNA determined that it would have the ultimate responsibility for financial management and therefore must maintain control over the program. Both boards approved full corporate merger as the vehicle of choice and proceeded to develop a joint resolution of intent to merge.

Clarification of the effect of merger on licensing, accreditation, and United Way affiliation was obtained. Blue Cross/Blue Shield and a bank trust department were consulted on the proposal. The approval of United Way, the National League for Nursing (NLN), the Michigan Department of Public Health, and the East Central Michigan Health Systems Agency (HSA) was obtained before further action was taken.

A timetable was developed cooperatively by the executive directors and legal consultants. The approval of the timetable, resolution, and plan for merger took place in January 1983. There were meetings of HOS volunteers and VNA staff with their respective boards to allay any concerns.

A governance chart and organizational charts were developed and negotiated. It was decided that hospice representation on the VNA board of directors was to be determined on the basis of budget ratios. In addition, necessary bylaw revisions and change in articles of incorporation that would meet each agency's approval had to be developed. Changes in job descriptions, space allocation, insurance coverage, and other considerations were reviewed, revised, and approved by appropriate standing committees of each board. At this time, meetings of both organizations' representatives were held frequently. Finally, at a joint board meeting held on March 29, 1983, the proposed bylaws, certificate of merger, and restated Articles of Incorporation were reviewed, and the resolution to merge was approved and signed by both parties. Approval by HOS membership occurred on the same day.

Hospice staff moved into the VNA office in March 1983, and the merger became official on May 1. Approval by the state of the merger occurred on May 31. The organizational chart and governance chart that were approved are shown on pages 195 and 196.

EPILOGUE

In retrospect, the merger of the two organizations resulted from the following causes:

1. The determination that the potential benefits of merger to the VNA outweighed the financial risks.

2. The commitment of the hospice board to continued fund raising for the program.

3. The commitment of the administrators and boards to compromise, when that was in the best interest of their respective organizations, and to maintain open minds in negotiations.

Organization Chart—VNA of Saginaw and Hospice of Saginaw

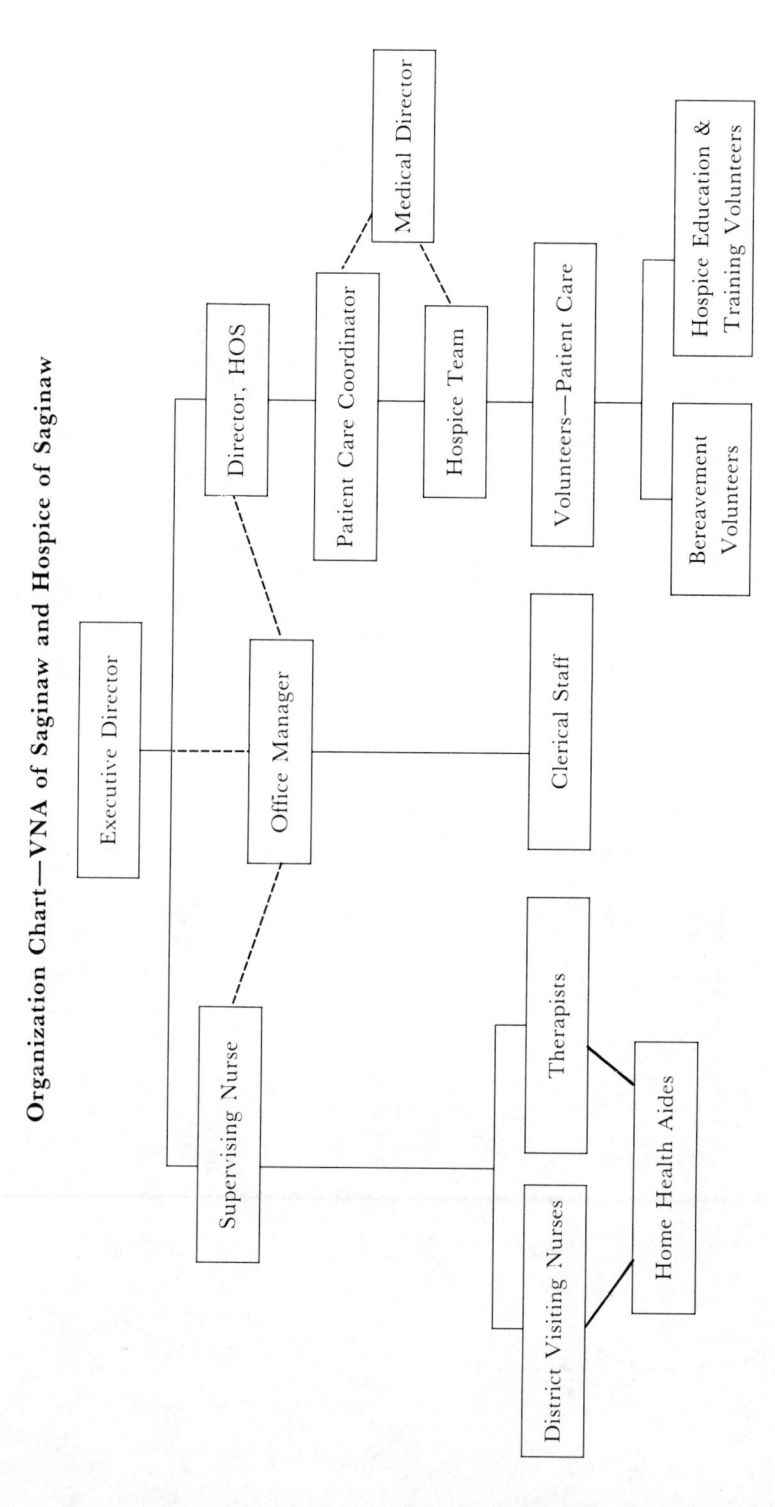

Governance Chart—VNA of Saginaw and Hospice of Saginaw

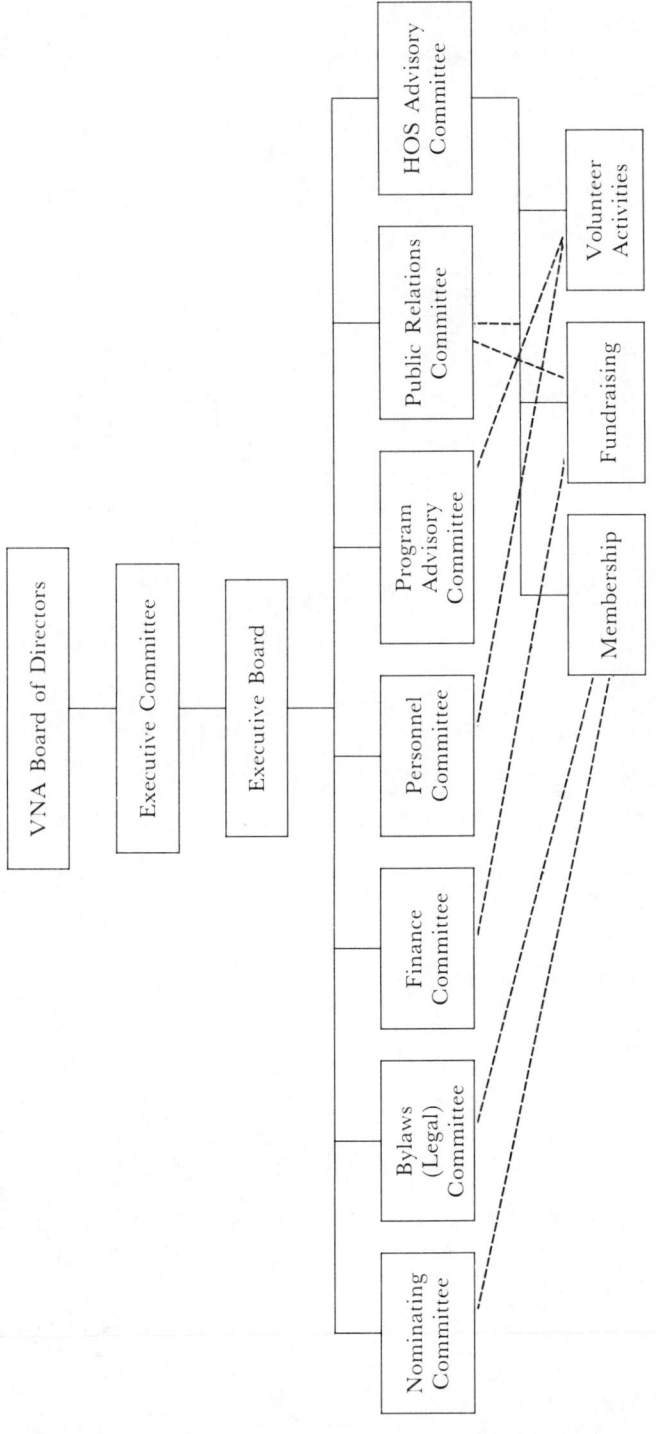

4. The help and encouragement of the community: United Way, the local HSA, physicians, and other agencies.
5. Legal consultation provided by an attorney respected by both organizations.
6. Willingness of both staffs to accept changes in their responsibilities.
7. The level of trust between staff and board in both organizations.

One of the crucial decisions involved which staff members would be retained by the VNA. Analysis of job functions within the VNA and hospice was completed by the executive directors and reviewed by the personnel committee of each board. Premerger HOS staff included the director, the patient care coordinator, a secretary, a bookkeeper, and home health aides. It was decided that the bookkeeper, home health aides, and secretary would duplicate VNA staff. However, vacancies existed for both home health aides and secretary at the VNA, and the bookkeeper was retained on an as-needed basis. Therefore, all staff members were assured of a position, though somewhat different from their position with HOS.

One year after merger the VNA reviewed the postmerger results. Hospice patient caseload had increased 35 percent, average length of stay was 36 days, and the cost per visit per family was reduced.

The merger strengthened the hospice program's political base by increasing physician recognition and United Way support and reestablishing the creditability of the program. Enlarged scope of services, improved continuity of care, and financial stability allowed the hospice program to develop its bereavement services and allowed the VNA the choice of seeking Medicare reimbursement for hospice services.

The growth of the total organization meant continuous change and adaptation for everyone concerned. Integration of staff continues to be a challenge. Both board and staff members must be persistent in closing the gap of "we" and "they." As time passes the gap continues to close, and hospice services through Hospice of Saginaw, a division of the VNA, continue to receive strong community support.

Case Example

Hospice Care, Inc.—A For-Profit Company

Mary Lou Gillespie

The development of the first free-standing for-profit hospice in this country was the result of the interest of several leaders in the hospice movement and the hospice Medicare regulations.

The idea began at the 1979 National Hospice Organization convention, in a rather prophetic speech given by Don Gaetz, who served as National Hospice Organization president in 1982-83 and is now a Hospice Care, Inc., vice-president:

> The greatest single obstacle to the development and even the survival of hospice in America is the lack of an adequate and equitable system to finance hospice care. Our high ideals will wither under the scorching reality that our programs cannot be financially viable. Our hospices will not live to adulthood and may even die in infancy if we cannot give the caregivers the tools and resources to render the total care that dying people need and deserve. This is one ill we cannot palliate. It must be cured in order for hospice to live.

Three years later, against overwhelming odds and in spite of opposition from organized health industry lobbies, Gaetz and his colleagues led an ad hoc coalition of hospices to victory in the legislative fight to establish hospice care as a Medicare-reimbursible service.

Many of the hospice leaders who were most deeply involved in drafting the hospice legislation and securing its approval by Congress and the president recognized that Medicare reimbursement for hospice service had to be quickly followed by the establishment of hospice in the private sector. Although Medicare beneficiaries constitute a significant majority of those needing hospice services, many people receive health coverage through employer-employee health plans. Hospice leaders were concerned that hospice service would primarily be available to the Medicare population. The Reverend Hugh Westbrook, president of Hospice Care, Inc., in a speech to the Michigan legislature, stated, "Hospices will face financial disaster and ethical paralysis unless and until we can eliminate the possibility of two-tiered care. There must not be well-reimbursed, comprehensive hospice services available to one class of patients in a hospice and far less available to non-Medicare patients."

Michigan became one of the first states to mandate hospice coverage in private health insurance plans. In addition, 39 Blue Cross plans have developed permanent or experimental hospice benefits, and several major commercial carriers were, as of mid-1984, nationally marketing the hospice benefit.

To those who first saw financial viability as a life-or-death issue for the hospice movement, the challenge of developing and maintaining a hospice program financially had not been resolved. Even though the national hospice reimbursement act had passed, the federal guidelines defined a payment methodology of prospective reimbursement that would make it financially difficult for hospices to survive. Prospectively set per-diem rates appeared to have the advantage of giving hospice caregivers more flexibility at the bedside. However, per-day costs were determined on an inadequate data base, and the rates were set so low that many of the nation's hospices, especially those with a daily patient census of 30 or fewer, could not provide all the services required by Medicare and break even on the per-diem rates.

Perhaps the greatest financial problem with prospectively set per-diem reimbursement rates is the lack of reimbursement for start-up costs. Unlike home health agencies, hospices are not permitted to capture developmental and start-up costs. Traditionally, hospices have been financed by community groups, religious organizations, foundations, United Ways, insurance carriers, and the Medicare systems. For most newly developing hospices the traditional routes will still be needed in spite of the new hospice benefit.

Gaetz and Westbrook proposed a plan to develop several new comprehensive hospice programs in areas with unmet needs and thus was born Hospice Care, Inc., an employee/corporate-owned organization designed to attract private financing sufficient to carry strategically placed hospices during the months and even years it might take until they reached a financially viable daily census. Gaetz and Westbrook found two banking firms and a small number of private individuals willing to risk money in venture capital in expectation of a potential after-tax return of 5-6 percent. The projected start-up time to reach 5-6 percent profitability was estimated to be four to five years.

To achieve the economies of scale necessary to spread costs over a large enough census, Hospice Care, Inc., developed an organizational model that minimizes overhead and places emphasis on using the reimbursement dollar for direct patient/family care. This required centralizing financial management, accounting, and billing all in one location, yet serving several hospices.

In order to reach census levels that would result in sufficient revenues to pay investors for their risks, Hospice Care, Inc., selectd initial sites where there were clearly unmet needs for hospice service: Miami, Florida; Ft. Lauderdale, Florida; and Dallas, Texas. Other sites under consideration are also in large Sunbelt cities. Hospice Care, Inc., operates two non-profit hospices in Florida and one for-profit hospice in Dallas, Texas. The organizational model of Dallas Hospice Care, Inc., is shown in Figure 2.2 on page 30.

The model, including three home care teams and one inpatient team, is designed to serve 650 patients per year. The patients and families are assigned to teams and the team directors coordinate all aspects of patient care, from admission to home care or inpatient care from weekly conference to discharge.

In planning the implementation phase in Dallas, Gaetz and Westbrook wanted experienced hospice staff to direct the local unit. They were able to hire a hospice management team that included an executive director, patient-care team director, volunteer director, and chaplain who had previously worked together in a local hospice program.

According to Westbrook, "Hospice Care, Inc., isn't a group of business people going into hospice. It's a group of hospice people using business skills and resources as a mechanism for fulfilling their long-time personal and professional objectives of finding ways to render hospice care competently and compassionately." Hospice Care, Inc., is a company with concerns for medically indigent patients and families and has committed $200,000 to their care annually, based on caring for 650 patients per year.

The Dallas Hospice Care, Inc., team moved into leased office space on January 16, 1984. Their initial plans included: (1) find physician applicants for medical director and team positions, (2) explore with hospital administrators the possibility of leasing space, (3) provide information on Dallas Hospice Care, Inc., to physicians, (4) provide information to health and social service organizations, (5) prepare policy and procedure manuals, and (6) prepare for Medicare certification and request hospice licensure.

After receiving approval to do business in Texas and completing basic policy and procedure manuals, Dallas Hospice Care, Inc., began accepting one or two patients per month. The first patient was admitted on February 21, 1984, and was cared for by the nurse team director, chaplain, and director of volunteers under the direction of the attending physician.

Negotiations for inpatient space began with a local hospital in February; however, the decision-making process of the hospital administration proved to be very lengthy. Therefore, Dallas Hospice Care, Inc., decided to develop temporary contracts with local hospitals until the inpatient unit opened. The first contact, with Gaston Episcopal Hospital, was signed in April 1984. The contract negotiations were facilitated by the hospital chaplain, who is a hospice advocate.

By early March, a medical director (an oncologist) was employed, and by the end of March the first team nurse, team physician, and marketing nurse were on staff. They were followed three weeks later by a second nurse, two home health aides, and a part-time social worker.

Dallas Hospice Care, Inc., was surveyed by Medicare on April 19-20, 1984, and received its Medicare provider number on July 20. At this writing we are the first and only hospice to be certified in Dallas under the new hospice Medicare regulations.

The average daily census in July was 25 patients per day, with a total of 70 patients served to date. Projections are for an average daily census of 70 by the end of 1984. Consistent with the values of its founders, Hospice Care, Inc., has a strong commitment to care for indigent patients. In its first six months of operation, for example, Dallas Hospice Care, Inc., has carried an indigent caseload of approximately 25 percent of its patient population. That is approximately twice the proportion of families who are below the poverty level in Dallas.

Our most serious problem so far has been that patients' physicians often do not have staff privileges at the hospital where we have contracted for inpatient facilities. This problem will likely be eliminated when we open our own inpatient facility and can approve physicians for admitting privileges. The only alternative would be to have contracts with all the major hospitals in Dallas; the coordination and monitoring of patient admissions required under those circumstances, however, and the provision of care plans to all the hospitals involved would be a challenge.

Dallas Hospice Care, Inc., brings to the city care that is individually coordinated and comprehensive in its services, as well as unique in its organizational structure (all permanent employees are given shares of stock in the company). Don Gaetz states, "While we come out of nonprofit backgrounds, we have found that one of the advantages of organizing as a proprietary entity is the ability to give ownership of the hospice, in very real and concrete terms, to those who render the care and do the work of caregiving. Nonprofit organizations can't provide that kind of ownership to employees. In nonprofit settings, people serve the institution and the institution just goes on and on. In the Hospice Care, Inc., for-profit setting, the success or failure of the hospice program is a very personal responsibility of every employee. We believe that makes for better hospice care and we believe it represents long-delayed participation and economic justice for hospice caregivers."

Case Example

Hospital-Based Hospice

Sister Dolores Castellano

As early as 1976, we at Mercy Hospital were looking at the needs of the terminally ill and their families. We found that general hospital regulations and big, busy inpatient units did not lend themselves to meeting these needs. The administration, committed to Mercy Hospital's philosophy of providing quality health care for the whole person, established a task force on the care of the dying to address the needs of the terminally ill and their families. Membership consisted of those who were interested in the subject and in working on the task force, including both department heads and staff. The administration appointed as chair, a person who had demonstrated great interest and concern for the terminally ill and their families. From the beginning of the study to the present, the task force has had strong approval and support from the administrator, maintained through open communication and reporting. Because the members of the task force came as volunteers interested in and concerned for the terminally ill, there was much participation and activity. Attendance at meetings was close to 100 percent; work assigned to subgroups was completed.

INITIAL RESEARCH AND PLANNING

Study and research were the first steps to be taken. The membership needed a broad knowledge base, including the state of the art in terminal care, the wider subject of death and dying, and what programs of care were available. We needed to assess what patients' needs were, what was being done, and what still needed to be done to meet the needs.

To assess the need for a terminal-care program on Long Island, we contacted institutions in and around New York City that cared for the terminally ill. Rosary Hill Home, in Hawthorne, New York, reported that one-quarter of the 300 patients they cared for each year came from Long Island. Other area hospitals did not report the number of patients they cared for who came from Long Island. A statistical study and joint audit was done by the social worker and pastoral counselor at Mercy Hospital to determine the total number of cancer inpatient deaths, the total terminal cancer patient days, the duration of terminal cancer hospitalizations, and the number of cancer deaths by department (e.g., medical, surgical, gynecological).

To gain an understanding of what was being done across the United States and Canada in the area of terminal care we did extensive reading, participated in workshops, and sought consultation. Consultations were obtained with Riverside Hospice, New Jersey; St. Luke's Hospice, New York; and the Shell of Hope, New York. In addition, over a period of two years we conducted three seminars at Mercy Hospital. The first was designed primarily for our own hospital staff. Because the staff members are responsible for the day-to-day care of patients and families, their knowledge, support, and participation would be necessary to the new program. We needed to provide opportunities for staff members to learn about the physical, emotional, social, and spiritual needs of the terminally ill. Seminars were subsequently offered to staff members of other health care institutions and the general public. The first two seminars consisted of two-hour sessions, held one evening a week for seven weeks. The last seminar, which was only five weeks long, was specifically on children and death. Among the guest speakers were physicians, social workers, nurses, clergymen, and families of hospice patients. The subject matter included death and dying, coping mechanisms, religious and cultural responses, and sources of support. The teaching methods included lectures, small-group discussion, audiovisual demonstrations, and role playing. Consultants were brought in from the Riverside Hospice in New Jersey, and other programs were contacted for information.

When we came to the conviction that a hospital-based hospice would answer our desire to better meet the needs of the terminally ill, we outlined goals and objectives. Our long-range goal was to set up a hospice at Mercy Hospital modeled after Saint Christopher's Hospice in London and the Palliative Care Service at Royal Victoria Hospital-McGill University in Montreal. Our immediate goal was to start up a pilot project that would demonstrate the need for and feasibility of hospice at Mercy Hospital, in Nassau County, New York. The objectives of the proposed program were to respond to the needs of individual terminally ill patients and their families; to fulfill the need for such a service in Nassau and Suffolk Counties; to provide a service that would maintain a quality of life that would be satisfying to the patient and family until death; to provide a model for other programs of high-quality care for the terminal patient and family; to serve as an education center for others by providing clinical and nonclinical programs; and to enable Mercy Hospital to express its philosophy of the dignity of each person in a concrete and comprehensive manner.

Questions and issues to be addressed at that time were: (1) identification of a working and successful model of care, (2) appropriateness of this model to our setting, (3) modifications that would have to be made, (4) cost, (5) location of the hospice unit within the hospital.

After much research, the program at Royal Victoria-McGill University, Montreal, was chosen as the model for us to study in depth and modify. Next we chose the setting, with the awareness that site selection would present new problems of its own. As health care providers are all aware, finances are almost always a problem. In addition to Medicare, Medicaid, and private insurance, we saw the need for additional funding. Therefore, we made grant proposals to the Long Island Cancer Council and to a private foundation. The decision to apply for a grant raised other administrative issues: (1) investment of staff time and money to write a grant, (2) investment of staff time and money to work with the granting organization, (3) uncertainty that the grant would be approved, (4) obligations imposed by the grant contract, and (5) restrictions set by the grant contract.

In the course of developing the program we recognized that it would be necessary to identify all those whom the program would affect, and those from whom we would need cooperation. Our goal would be to obtain support through exchange of information and encouragement of participation in planning. We needed to provide information and seek suggestions and comments. The program had to be defined concretely and specifically, and why the program was needed and what we hoped to accomplish had to be stated. The groups we needed to communicate with were the board of directors, the department heads, physicians, nursing staff, and the community. Meetings were held with the department heads and physicians. Presentations were given at board of directors' meetings. The three seminars on the care of the dying were held for Mercy Hospital personnel and the community.

At the same time we were in the planning phase of our hospice program, *Newsday,* the local newspaper, asked for a story on how we cared for the dying and their families at Mercy Hospital. Their knowledge of the way a specific case was handled at Mercy through our pastoral care department motivated the request, and the reporters were impressed with what they saw at the hospital. When they heard about our plans for a hospice program, they requested a further interview. This gave us an opportunity to give information to the general public, not only through *Newsday* but also through feature articles in the *Long Island Catholic* and various other publications.

In addition to the group meeting with department heads, meetings with individual department heads were held. This was considered necessary because the philosophy of the hospice would necessarily demand administrative changes. For example, 24-hour visiting privileges would create a need for additional housekeeping: the living room would be used continuously, and the coffee corner would require extra clean-up work. Because we wanted to create a cheerful atmosphere, we ordered floral sheets and pillow cases, which would cause a change in the laundry sorting and delivery systems. The area chosen did not have piped-in oxygen or suction equipment; therefore we would need the cooperation of the cardiopulmonary and central services departments to obtain oxygen tanks and portable suction equipment when needed. Controlling pain is given high priority in hospice care, so we needed the cooperation and the support of the pharmacy. The admission procedure for hospice patients would be different from that for other patients. Because we involved staff members in the planning of the program, we had exceptional cooperation. The laundry agreed to use fitted sheets even though this required a change in laundry procedure; the pharmacy developed a service to distribute medications to hospice patients on an outpatient basis. They also circulated a newsletter on pain medication and pain control.

Issues and Problems

The area chosen for the hospice presented a problem. We were to use 12 beds of an existing 47-bed unit and share the desk area, medication area, personnel lockers, and so forth. Thus two separate nursing staffs with two different philosophies or approaches to care were to coexist on the same unit. The aim of the hospice administration was to gain a welcome on the unit, present the change in as nonthreatening a manner as possible, and build a positive relationship between the two staffs.

While planning and organizing was in process in our local area, we recognized that we must keep informed about developments in the hospice movement on the state and national levels. We kept up and extended our contacts with other programs in both the planning and operational phases. We attended the first national meeting of the National Hospice Organization (NHO) and became a provisional member with voting privileges. We felt that our NHO membership would keep us informed about this new and fast-developing movement, as well as giving us help in setting standards and criteria. Through this organization we have exchanged information with colleagues and gained support.

We became involved at the state level by attending meetings in the state capital directed by the Health Systems Management office. These meetings served as an arena to gain information, to give feedback to the state on local concerns and happenings, and to get a sense of direction.

Our interactions with some of the supporting systems raised additional issues and problems. At the NHO meeting in Washington in 1978, standards and criteria for hospice were presented. There was much discussion, misinterpretation, and confusion. It was evident that all participants did not share a common perspective. Some were already involved in delivery of care, others were in the planning phase, others the study phase, others were only interested in hospice, while still others represented third-party payors and various organizations. To make the discussions more complex, there was a varied geographical representation. What is good in a rural area may not be good in a large city, and vice versa. While some areas need new organizations and agencies to deliver services, others need to foster cooperation and coordination among existing services and agencies. Laws vary from state to state. Although this type of gathering and discussion is informative, it can promote confusion, hard feelings, and misunderstanding. We in the hospice movement were experiencing growing pains. However, we were grateful that the National Hospice Organization set as its primary goal to preserve the philosophy of hospice and to maintain standards of care.

Accreditation became an issue. Who is responsible for the accreditation of hospices? Which groups need accreditation? Why should an accredited hospital or home care agency need further accreditation? For example, hospitals accredited by the JCAH questioned the need of additional accreditation. Should existing agencies undergo the same review as those trying to create new agencies? Should existing accredited agencies be reviewed after program expansion?

Another issue was uncertainty on how various state governments and the federal government would classify hospice beds for reimbursement purposes. The philosophy of hospice care is that care must be carried out on a continuum: regardless of the patient's physical location (home, hospital-based hospice, nursing-home-based hospice, freestanding hospice), the patient and family's physical, emotional, social, and spiritual needs must be cared for. Because a patient's needs change during the course of the illness, each setting plays a significant role in the care of the terminally ill and should be used as needed to meet the needs of patients and families. Each setting should be evaluated for reimbursement and classification according to the services rendered.

Another issue for the administrator of a new program is the question of responsibility to spread the good news, so that a philosophy you believe in can spread and grow. New programs need continual study, evaluation, and development. They must function before they can be evaluated. Time spent on consultation and public relations takes away from time available for administration, development, further study, and planning.

The issue of cost containment, so prominent in health care today, conflicts with program development. A new program generally means more money must be expended, at least initially. However, it is important not to compromise on the essentials of a program. Sometimes this can be avoided by implementing the program in stages. If you find that you must compromise on essential components of the program, it is better to wait until the compromise is no longer necessary. An example of a serious compromise would be in the number of nurses needed to carry out the plan. Nursing is integral to the hospital-based hospice. The nurse must be able to deliver excellent care and be able to care for the family as well as the patient. A key element in delivery of hospice care is time—time for the nursing staff to care for the patient and family, time to make each moment rich for the patient, time to enhance life and prepare for death. If the number of nurses on staff is such that the philosophy cannot be carried out, then delay the implementation of the plan.

In addition to all these considerations, other internal and external restrictions can create problems. Some internal restrictions we considered were the space available to carry out the program and the support services available (dietary, pharmacy, etc.). Space and decor are of primary concern to the inpatient hospice. Space is needed for unlimited visitors, patient and family conferences, staff conferences, recreation, and dining. The hospice program must be independent, physically apart from other patient areas, because independence allows for creativity and flexibility. Serious consideration should be given to the number of inpatient beds that will be available. Besides causing frustration, having too few beds may result in a program that is too small to be cost effective. On the other had, compromises in service can occur when a program is too large.

Among the external restrictions that we faced were those related to our Long Island Cancer Council grant agreement. Only patients with cancer in specific sites could be admitted to the program. The local Health Systems Agency and state health department were involved in review of the application, modifying the program, and giving final approvals.

Restrictions do not necessarily have a negative effect: sometimes they free us by forcing us to streamline our programs and distinguish essential from nonessential elements. Sometimes they force us to focus on the goal and give less attention to fringes. Sometimes they force us to set priorities and question our values. The following were established as our priorities: establishing a hospice team and choosing nursing staff, hiring a volunteer coordinator and a program secretary, and determining the physical location. It was decided to leave the development of a formal bereavement program until last.

IMPLEMENTATION

Once the research and education phases were coming to completion and appropriate groups and individuals had been included in our projections for change, concrete planning for implementation of the hospice program began. A target date of September 5, 1978, was set for services to begin. The organization of an interdisciplinary team, staff selection and orientation, the establishment of a temporary inpatient unit, and the formulation of policies and procedures all had to be accomplished before that time.

The interdisciplinary team was formed of members of the task force on the care of the dying who had researched and developed the concept of hospice care for Mercy Hospital. The hospice team was to consist of a medical director, program director, head nurse, pastoral counselor, nutritionist, social worker, volunteer coordinator, and home care coordinator. The initial team was composed of myself (a nursing care coordinator), two physicians (a family practitioner and a surgeon), a pastoral counselor (the head of the department of pastoral care), a social worker, the secretary of the pastoral care department (the future volunteer coordinator), and a nutritionist. We had our first meeting in January 1978. The minutes of the first meetings show that we began to form ourselves into a team. All team members were asked to describe their ideas of what their roles would be in the proposed hospice program. Clinical concerns were discussed and researched at this time. The nutritionist provided materials on nutritional needs of advanced cancer patients. Pain control methods and types of medication were described. A site for the inpatient unit was chosen. Recognizing the need to keep the medical staff and general hospital leadership involved in the plans and activities of the hospice team, we sought membership on the hospital patient care committee and attended medical staff meetings.

Staff Selection and Orientation

In May 1978, the team began discussing steps to be followed in opening the hospice. Selection and training of staff and the formulation of policies and procedures were the first areas to be addressed. In June 1978, we posted in the hospital notices of available positions in the new program. We did not ask staff of an existing nursing unit to assume responsibility for the new program, because we felt strongly that those who should care for the terminally ill and their families would be volunteers. This could not be a mandatory assignment. Once hospital employees had been given the opportunity to apply, an advertisement was placed in the newspapers and selection of staff members began.

The initial interview consisted of the exchange of information and completion of a questionnaire. Since the hospice concept was new not only to Mercy but to the public in general, the proposed hospice program had to be explained in detail. The applicants were asked to tell us why they had applied, what they believed they had to offer, and what they hoped to gain for themselves. The purpose of the questionnaire was to find out what special talents and interests the applicants had and to gain insight into their feelings about death and dying and the terminally ill. Criteria used in selection were the applicant's previous experience (at least two years' medical-surgical experience in a hospital was required), the results of the interview, and the questionnaire. Those who met all the qualifications but had experienced the death of a person close to them within the last year were not accepted. They were asked to reapply if they were still interested after at least one year had elapsed since the death.

By the end of August 1978, screening and selection of hospice nursing staff, secretarial staff, and volunteer coordinator were completed. A one-week orientation program for the nursing staff was given the week of September 4, 1978. The entire nursing staff attended the 30-hour program. The objectives of the orientation were to familiarize the staff with the goals and services of the Mercy Hospital Hospice and to provide education on cancer, the dying patient, and treatment modalities. The overall goal of the orientation program was to establish an atmosphere in which the staff could begin to form a cohesive group.

During the first hour of the orientation, each staff member was introduced to the group. Each person's special talents, as identified during the interviews, were described. Each member of the hospice team was introduced, and each person described the role he or she would play in the delivery of care and in directing the program. There were lectures on pain and pain control, family crisis and intervention, coping mechanisms, death and dying, cancer treatment, and comfort measures. A session was devoted to self-awareness about death and dying.

The Volunteer Program

During June and July 1978 the volunteer coordinator organized the volunteer components of the program. She obtained volunteers through referrals from church organizations as a result of community awareness. Prospective volunteers filled out a written application, had a personal interview, and completed an orientation program. By August 19, 1978, the orientation program was in progress. The program consisted of seven 3-hour sessions given by members of the hospice team. The sessions included an introduction to the program, personal orientation, the emotional, social, physical, and spiritual aspects of care, practical procedures, and a summary session. There were 45 volunteers ready to begin work in September 1978.

Each volunteer made a commitment to serve for at least one year and to provide 16 hours of service per month. These hours would include time spent at support groups, education sessions, and the hospice family mass and coffee hour. Volunteers were assigned to the hospice unit on an hourly basis starting at 7 a.m. and ending at 9 p.m. Each tour of service would be for three hours. Activities would include assisting the nurse at the bedside, running errands, sitting and talking with families in the living room, attending to the coffee corner, and providing companionship to patients. Other volunteers would be on call from 11 p.m. to 7 a.m. to sit with frightened or confused patients when needed. Another group of volunteers would make home visits, while still others would do office work or take responsibility for the monthly hospice family mass and coffee hour.

The volunteer coordinator, sensitive to the needs of the volunteers, planned to hold twice-monthly support group meetings (both day and evening). Opportunities for more in-depth learning were planned, including monthly educational meetings using guest speakers. Among the educational programs was one on the Red Cross home care program. Mechanisms for communication between the volunteer coordinator and volunteers were set up. Volunteers would keep a weekly log to document their activities, comments, and feelings. The volunteer coordinator would distribute a monthly newsletter to keep the volunteers informed of events, activities, and general information. In addition, the volunteer coordinator would be available in person and by phone.

Home Care Services

Since we were committed to keeping our patients at home with their families for as long as possible, we had to plan for home care services. We did not have an organized home care department at the hospital, nor did we have the possibility of setting up our own home care department or agency. Our goals were to provide services to patients and families, to be cost effective, and to work within the existing health care system. We had enjoyed good working relationships with the certified home health agencies in Nassau and Suffolk counties in the past and looked forward to a continued working relationship. Joint meetings were held with the directors of the Nursing Sisters Home Visiting Service, Incorporated, the Visiting Home Health Services of Nassau, and the Nassau County Department of Health. We at hospice described our goals, what we were doing, what we hoped to accomplish, and what we identified as needs. As a result of the meetings, transfer agreements were made with the agencies for home care of our hospice patients and educational programs were planned for the staff of the home care agencies. The Nursing Sisters Home Visiting Service would provide a public health nurse to assume the role of hospice home care coordinator. She would be a member of the hospice team, would act as a liaison between the hospital and the home health agencies, and would work with the hospice inpatient staff, patients, and families to prepare the patients to go home. Once the patient was at home, she would make follow-up calls and home visits for assessment and ongoing coordination.

As a result of our grant with the Long Island Cancer Council, we were able to derive benefits for our patients when at home. The subcontractors of the Long Island Cancer Council worked together for the benefit of patients having cancer. The Visiting Homemaker Service, Inc., of Huntington, New York, a subcontractor of the Long Island Cancer Council, would supply homemaker and home health aide services for our patients.

Bereavement Program

The bereavement program was developed in stages. It was decided that the families would receive bereavement follow-up for a period of at least one year after the patient died. When possible, members of the hospice team, nurses, or volunteers would attend wakes and funerals. The initial phase of the program included follow-up phone calls to the bereaved on a two-week, six-week, three-month, six-month, nine-month, and twelve-month schedule made by the nurses, pastoral counselor, or social worker. Forms were developed on which to record the name of the person contacted, the date, an assessment of the coping or grief response, and the conversation that took place. These reports were brought to the weekly team meetings and discussed.

On a monthly basis, invitations were extended to family and friends of deceased patients to attend the hospice family mass and coffee hour. This was an informal gathering for all associated with the hospice program. The volunteers assumed the responsibility for this service.

The second phase of the bereavement program was the development of groups. Members of the hospice team and inpatient nursing staff expressed interest in the development of a group and in running the group. The expertise of a psychiatric social worker was obtained to provide information and direction. Group leadership skills, group dynamics, family coping mechanisms, and responses to loss were among the topics discussed. Extensive reading on grief and bereavement was done. The mechanics of forming the group, group size, frequency of meetings, composition of the group, and the type of group werre discussed. Postmeeting consultation sessions were planned with the psychiatric social worker, to review the group process and content and to obtain guidance.

It was decided that two weeks after the death of a patient, an introductory letter would be sent to the family describing the bereavement group. Four weeks later an invitation would be sent, advising the family of the group schedule and asking whether they would participate. The group size would be limited to 15 people. Meetings would be held twice monthly outside the hospital. Only family members of hospice patients would be accepted. The groups would be open-ended and participants could attend at will.

Because not all people choose to participate in groups, we realized that one-to-one bereavement support was needed as well. The pastoral counselor and social worker were to set up individual counseling sessions as needed.

Policies and Procedures

The development of job descriptions and policies and procedures went on concurrently with formation of the hospice team, screening and selection of staff and volunteers, and the development of the orientation and bereavement programs. Job descriptions were developed for the director of hospice, the medical director, the social worker, the home care coordinator, the nutritionist, the sister chaplain, the head nurse, the primary nurse, the volunteer coordinator, and the program secretary. All members of the team had direct input into all job descriptions before they were finalized.

The following definition was formulated to describe the hospice program at Mercy Hospital: "The Hospice is established as a comprehensive program, including home care and inpatient care, for patients with a terminal illness and their families. It has as its goal to provide comfort through symptom control, hope based upon being well cared for, and a quality of life that is satisfactory to the patient and family until death. It is a therapeutic environment designed from the patients' point of view, with an at-home feeling. It is an effort to meet the needs of the patient with a terminal illness in a more appropriate manner."

The hospice team was responsible for writing and approving policies and procedures. Policies were developed for admissions, admission criteria, discharge, treatment guidelines, visiting guidelines, home care, bereavement services, the bereavement group, volunteer orientation, volunteer educational requirements, volunteer assignments, volunteer supervision, and the advisory committee. Procedures were developed to coincide with the policies on admissions, visiting guidelines, home care, and bereavement services.

Our first policies and procedures were developed to clarify and support program goals and objectives. For example, the policy on visiting guidelines states that the purpose of visiting in the hospice is to foster relationships and prevent feelings of anxiety and isolation. Opportunity for friends and family to spend time with the patients can serve to lessen the stresses of the illness for both patient and visitor. Participation in patient care fosters communication and the expression of feeling, and helps to prepare the survivors for the impending loss. In addition, family members need time for themselves to reestablish themselves and become refreshed. Therefore, the procedures allow visiting on a 24-hour basis, visitors can stay overnight, family participation in patient care is encouraged, children can visit, and every Monday is a visitor-free day.

Outside Contacts: Education, Funding, and Research

During the planning phase of the hospice program we realized that we would need to continue to increase our knowledge of death and dying, gain assistance in team functioning and interaction, and recognize areas of growth and stress, both personally and as a group. Seminars were arranged through the Shell of Hope, an institute for research and education about American attitudes toward death. A weekend seminar for volunteers, eight 2-hour sessions over a period of 10 weeks for nursing staff, and four 5-hour sessions for the hospice team were planned. These seminars were offered three to six months after the hospice program became operational.

An initial meeting with the Long Island Cancer Council to express interest in obtaining a grant was held on August 1, 1977. We were encouraged to write a formal letter of request and to begin to write a proposal. Our initial letter of request was dated October 11, 1977. The grant application was submitted by mid-1978, and a contract was signed in early 1979. The grant was for two years and would fund the salaries of the hospice project director, program secretary, and volunteer coordinator. It also provided funding for an expanded formal education component. In return, we would provide twice the amount of the grant in the form of services in kind, to be provided by volunteers and the volunteer services of professionals. Our first bimonthly report was given on October 31, 1978. At that time, we had served 27 patients and their families, experienced 7 patient deaths, and provided 236 lay volunteer and 202 professional volunteer hours of service.

In 1979 the Mery Hospital Hospice, along with 14 other programs, was selected for the New York State Hospice Demonstration Program. We and 11 other programs were able to establish services and supply data to the New York State Department of Health for inclusion in a study of the need for hospice within the health care system. In 1982 the Office of Health Systems Management published *An Analysis and Evaluation of the New York State Hospice Demonstration Program*. Since 1979 we have been required to submit program statistics and financial reports. We have participated in a survey of primary caregivers and have had consultation and support from the Office of Health Systems Management.

A requirement for participation in the demonstration was the establishment of the hospice as an autonomous program within the hospital. The hospice director reports directly to the hospital's chief executive officer and director of nursing. The hospice program secretary, volunteer coordinator, head nurse, and members of the formal hospice team report directly to the hospice director. A hospice advisory committee to the hospital board of directors was established. It is composed of representatives from hospice organizations, consumer representatives, and other appropriate persons not directly affiliated with the hospice. The hospice director is responsible for reporting to the Long Island Cancer Council and the State of New York, providing administrative leadership and coordination for the hospice program, providing for quality assurance, taking an active role in education and community relations, acting as a consultant for colleagues, and participating in New York and National Hospice Organization meetings.

RECENT DEVELOPMENTS

Since our establishment as a hospice in 1978, we have forged ahead with program development and expansion. On May 16, 1981, we dedicated our hospice inpatient unit. We moved from temporary quarters on an existing inpatient unit to a rebuilt, specially designed segregated unit. Later in the year we obtained approval to expand our inpatient capacity to 18 beds. This resulted in the need to increase staff size.

As of April 1984 we have served 825 families. Our hospice team has met on a weekly basis for the purpose of continued planning, implementation, and evaluation of patient and family care and of the total program. The bereavement group has met twice each month with an average attendance of 12 persons. An average of 45 bereavement calls are made each month. The hospice family mass and coffee hour has an average monthly attendance of 120 family members, volunteers, and staff. We have an average of 100 volunteers who provide approximately 1,800 hours of service per month. We receive approximately 100 individual donations per month, accompanied by letters of appreciation and indebtedness.

Presently, hospice programs like ours are in a critical situation. The requirements of Medicare certification pose serious problems. Medicare requires the hospice to provide 80 percent of its services in the home and only 20 percent in the inpatient setting. Our experience over the past six years is in conflict with this requirement. Our patient population has been a very ill and dependent one, and patients have spent the majority of their time in the inpatient setting. The average length of stay in the program for the six-month period from November 1983 to April 1984 was 30 days. During the same time period, the average length of inpatient stay was 17 days. Thus our patients would exceed the Medicare inpatient benefit. The hospice benefit under Medicare allows for a maximum of 210 days of care, but it is clear that we are receiving patients only during the final phase of their illness when they require intensified care and the cost of care rises markedly. In spite of our patient population and the type of care we render, however, the New York State Hospice Demonstration Program analysis revealed that all the demonstration programs were less costly than traditional care. We are concerned that hospice programs will hesitate to admit this group of terminally ill patients because of financial restrictions imposed by the Medicare regulations.

We are committed to providing hospice care to these patients and their families. Eight years ago we were convinced that the terminally ill and their families should receive priority treatment. They should not be dumped on busy medical-surgical units to compete with fresh postoperative patients and new medical admissions for care. Nor should they be on the bottom of a list when in need of an inpatient bed. Our experience has taught us that our conviction eight years ago was a sound conviction. The long hours of study and planning that resulted in the Mercy Hospital hospice program were worth the effort. We will continue the struggle to deliver their rightful care to the terminally ill and their families.

Case Example

Long-Term-Care – Based Hospice Program

Sister M. Karen McNally

One might imagine that starting a hospice care program in a well-established long-term-care facility would be a relatively simple task, given the accessibility of professional and medical services and the availability of inpatient beds. To those uninitiated in administering a hospice program, these understandably suggest readiness and adequate preparation. Having recently completed this task, I can reflect and comment on some of the many steps involved, as well as some of the challenges and pitfalls, since ours were certainly not entirely unique. Above all, I want to convey the sense of deep satisfaction and gratitude that an administrative staff feels as it witnesses the metamorphosis of a plan from its conception to its articulation to its implementation as a vital program providing care, concern, and loving support to dying persons and their families.

Some background about our institution and its surrounding facilities may promote a better understanding of the process of transforming our dream into a reality. The Cardinal Shehan Center for the Aging is located in Towson, Maryland. Stella Maris, the oldest and largest component, was opened in 1953 and now has 438 licensed long-term-care beds. Expansion since 1953, both in buildings and in services, has resulted in the newly named complex, the Cardinal Shehan Center. In addition to Stella Maris, the Center now includes Saint Elizabeth Hall, a HUD-202 apartment building with 200 units, 100 of which are Section 8 subsidized; Blessed Sacrament Residence, a Section 8 pilot project in Baltimore City for 16 older persons; and Saint John Hall Long Crandon, a home for 11 retired priests. An outreach program provides pastoral care to a nursing home in the city in addition to services for those waiting to be admitted into one of our residential programs.

When it first opened in 1953, Stella Maris, called Stella Maris Hospice at that time, was a retirement house for well elderly persons. As the residents grew older, nursing care was expanded to meet their needs. At that time, the word "hospice" in the title signified a stopping-off or resting place along the journey of life. As society's view of the institutionalized elderly changed and as Medicare and Medicaid guidelines for reimbursement became stricter, the character of the facility changed from a retirement home to a skilled and intermediate-level nursing home. With this change came the further development of already existing professional services, as well as the addition of new ones to provide medical, nursing, dietetic, social work, physical therapy, occupational therapy, speech therapy, pharmacy, and pastoral care services.

Well-developed professional services were strong influences in our decision to provide hospice care, because we had the components of an interdisciplinary team already in place. In spite of these positive features, two historical factors later proved to be liabilities in our marketing efforts for hospice care. The first was the fact that the facility was known as Stella Maris *Hospice* for 29 years before we officially started hospice care, and the second was its public image as an institution that primarily served the elderly.

CONCEPTION OF THE HOSPICE CARE PROGRAM

In 1979, the long-range planning committee of the Cardinal Shehan Center, composed of some board and some staff members, began to look at future needs. They identified hospice care and home care as two components on the continuum of care that we had not addressed. These components of care were identified after the committee reflected on the following sentence from the institution's mission statement: "The Cardinal Shehan Center for the Aging, with Stella Maris being the primary resource facility, provides a Christian atmosphere for comprehensive services, responding to the changing needs of persons within the boundaries of the Archdiocese of Baltimore." Hospice care was not contrary to our mission but an extension of our care for those far along on the journey of life. Hospice care would extend these services to the patient's home and to those under 65 years of age, and would be directed toward supporting those in the final months of their journey.

PLANNING OF THE HOSPICE CARE PROGRAM

After the long-range plan was approved, the task of developing a strategy to implement hospice care was transferred to a working staff group. Since staff members of all disciplines would be involved in delivering hospice care, it was considered important that all disciplines be represented on the planning committee. In addition, some staff members asked to serve on the committee because of personal interest in the project. The chairperson welcomed anyone who wished to participate, which resulted in a committee of 33 members, which proved to be unwieldy. A great deal of conflict resulted from our attempts to determine the optimum size for this group. On the one hand, it was felt that the advantages of including a large group in a working task force would be twofold. It would serve to introduce a significant portion of the staff to the idea of hospice care, and it would involve all the professional disciplines in the development of the program from the early planning stages, thus effecting interest and ownership. On the other hand, a committee with 33 members had tremendous disadvantages. First, it was difficult to organize such a large group. Communication and attendance both created problems. The third and most significant problem was that we were not able to include all those who had participated in the planning process in the staff of the new program when it was implemented. This proved to be a true hardship for some staff members when the new program opened.

However, in this large group, representatives of all departments began to develop a plan for a hospice care program at Stella Maris. The initial step was to identify the tasks that had to be completed before we could start the program. We assigned responsibility for completion of these tasks to staff volunteers and set an expected date of completion for each task. The statements of assignments included the main goal, steps toward its accomplishment, person or persons responsible for completing each task, and the date by which each task had to be completed. This served to concretize the overall goal of establishing the program by making it seem feasible. Second, it made the subgroups a more workable size, and third, it made all members responsible for some part of the project.

We then formed a steering committee of three members whose function was to monitor progress, identify potential problems, and motivate and assist the subgroups as they worked to complete their assignments.

The tasks themselves included research, definition of the program, development of the home care program, writing departmental guidelines and admission and medical protocols, investigation of legal and regulatory issues, selection of hospice team members, setting up educational procedures, making the program known to the community, and developing evaluation tools. These tasks were carried out simultaneously with the support and assistance of the steering committee. First, we carried out research to give us the information necessary for later decision making. Areas of research included the strengths and weaknesses of existing hospice programs, the need for additional hospice care in our area, and possible sources of funding. It was important to us to study other programs to determine if a long-term-care–based program could be a true hospice and also to avoid repeating the mistakes that others had made. Various staff members visited hospice programs and noted the strong points of each. Another staff member began work on possible sources of funding to cover the start-up costs of the program.

The second task was to define the hospice care program that *we* wanted to create. The staff members who worked in this subgroup were responsible for putting on paper our definition of hospice care, philosophy of hospice care, and initial goals and objectives of the program. Although this was difficult to do, it made us define exactly what we wanted our program to be and do. It also made us decide what elements we did *not* want in our program.

Initial goals and objectives adopted for the hospice program were as follows:

Goal I To develop a nursing-home – based model for hospice care, including both inpatient and home-health aspects.

Objectives

To submit grant proposals in 1982 to obtain funding for the home care start-up costs.

To develop plans with the Renovations Committee to convert hall 400 South into a 13-bed inpatient pain management and hospice care unit.

To develop staffing patterns for the inpatient and home care programs.

To hire qualified staff to carry out the above-defined programs.

To obtain support and reimbursement from appropriate third-party payors, such as Medicare, Medicaid, and private carriers.

As we were working on the above objectives we simultaneously and quickly began effecting four of the five, leaving the hiring process until the later stages of development.

Goal II To enhance the quality of life, security, and comfort of terminally ill persons who wish to die at home.

Objectives

To provide intermittent skilled nursing services (two nurses and one aide) during the first year of this program's operation, beginning January 1983.

To provide the services of an interdisciplinary team of professionals and volunteers as necessary for terminally ill home care patients.

To provide support to families and significant others during this period of stress by assisting them in obtaining needed services and equipment.

To provide bereavement services to the family and significant others.

Goal III To emphasize the following key elements in this nursing-home – based model of hospice care.

  A. Pain management and symptom control.

  B. Flexibility, ease, and continuity in utilization of the dual elements in the program, allowing for both home care and inpatient services according to the patient's need at various stages.

  C. Patient control in the development of the plan of care.

  D. Cost effectiveness combined with excellence in delivery of care.

Objectives

To develop a nursing staff proficient in pain assessment and management.

To have home care and inpatient interdisciplinary staffs meet together weekly to coordinate the care of all patients in the hospice care program.

To focus the plan of care around the patient's opinions and needs.

To monitor costs and determine cost-effective methods to provide quality care.

The third task in the plan was to develop the home care component, since home care is of primary importance in the concept of hospice and Stella Maris did not previously have a home care program. After months of debating whether or not to contract for home care services, our final decision was to start our own program. Our reasoning was based on two premises: (1) we wanted to ensure the quality of the home care component, since it is primary to hospice care, and (2) we did not feel that establishing a new program would duplicate existing services in the area. After this decision was approved by our administration and the board, the next task of the home care group was to define the home care program's relationship with the existing facility. The decision was made and approved to establish a licensed, certified home-health agency that would serve as a base for the hospice care program and also serve the local community with routine home health care.

The fourth task to be accomplished as part of the plan to implement hospice care was to define departmental guidelines for medicine, nursing, social work, staff development, volunteer services, programs and activities, pharmacy, physical therapy, and pastoral care. The subgroup working on this task involved members of each of these departments in defining their service and its protocols in the delivery of hospice care. This proved to be most effective in the later implementation of the program, since it required the members of each department to think through the delivery of service in relation to the philosophy and goals and objectives of the hospice program. It also set the stage for the interdisciplinary team function. Staff members did an excellent job of developing these guidelines and thus demonstrated an understanding of the delivery of hospice care relative to their respective departments. These guidelines, later called service plans, were all written in a consistent format and contained the name of the department, its philosophy of hospice care, and responsibilities in delivery of care.

The fifth task, assigned to yet another subgroup, was to develop appropriate protocols for admissions to the program and for attending physician services. Because they were very broad, the admissions protocols that were developed have remained relatively unchanged. The admissions policy, however, which is more specific, has been revised numerous times in the two years since it was written. Experience made us aware of our need to redefine our catchment area. This had originally been defined as a 30-*mile* driving radius. Because of the difference in city and highway driving times, we have since changed that to a 20-*minute* driving radius. In addition, for Title 6 requirements, we have also eliminated age specifications from the admissions policy.

Attending physician protocols were included in the list of documents to be developed for two reasons. First, hospice treatment is different from curative treatment, and second, working with attending physicians through home care was a new relationship for us. Our experience has proved that these protocols are invaluable in the routine delivery of care.

The sixth task to be completed prior to the implementation of our program was clarification of legal and regulatory issues. These include certificate of need, licensure, certification, and reimbursement. Since these were somewhat technical, they were done by me, as the institution's associate administrator. With the assistance of our legal counsel, all of the issues were resolved. A certificate of need (CON) was not necessary at the time for our home health program, because it was part of an existing licensed health care facility. That law has since changed in the state of Maryland, and all new home health agencies now require a CON. Since we were using existing beds, we did not require a CON for inpatient beds. We did, however, keep the state planning agency informed of what we were doing. Currently, there is no licensure mechanism for hospice in our state; thus our inpatient beds and home health agency are part of our licensed long-term-care facility. Both, however, have been certified by Medicare for reimbursement purposes.

Simultaneously, we were working with Blue Cross of Maryland to participate in their hospice pilot program. Our home care program was approved first, and later the inpatient unit. It took much longer to get the inpatient unit approved for reimbursement because we are not a hospital nor did we fit any of the existing models for hospice care. Convinced of the effectiveness of our home care and inpatient components under a central administration that could integrate hospice treatment and philosophy, we were eager to work with groups such as Blue Cross to demonstrate that our program could provide the highest quality service while being cost effective for the third-party payor. Not surprisingly, a significant commitment of time and completion of detailed paperwork preceded approval for our participation in the pilot program.

The seventh task of the development phase of the hospice program was to select the hospice team and begin its work. As we were concurrently carrying out the other tasks in the plan, we realized that this step was more applicable to the immediate implementation stage. Thus we tabled it for later attention.

The eighth part of the plan was to develop educational materials and programs for staff, potential hospice families, volunteers, and board members. The responsibility for developing most of these was entrusted to our staff development coordinator and her assistants. A special week was set aside during which a series of programs was offered each day. Panel discussions were held on the interdisciplinary team concept, and this topic was also offered as the subject of our regular weekly unit conferences. Family members of patients who had died in our long-term-care facility presented a panel on their personal experiences of the loss of a loved one. The theological and psychological aspects of suffering, loss, and grief were presented in special lectures with guest speakers. The week ended with a special liturgical function for the sick and terminally ill. The events of this week not only served to educate all staff and board members about the concept of hospice care but also to help staff members realize how they could implement aspects of hospice care in the long-term-care section of the Center.

The ninth task, the development of a public relations strategy, was accomplished by our director of public relations. She developed a schedule and planned content for news releases, articles in local newspapers, a brochure, and various speaking engagements with civic and church groups. This has been an ongoing effort and has since expanded to include luncheons for social workers engaged in discharge planning. These luncheons include informal discussions and question-and-answer periods in which key team members have explained the operations of our program.

The final component of the initial plan was the development of a mechanism for evaluation. A plan for later evaluation was required for state certification of the home care program and also for approval by insurance carriers. In the plan developed, both utilization review and professional advisory committees participate in the evaluation process. Simultaneously with the development of the evaluation plan, we coordinated the development of job descriptions for all members of the team, the organizational chart for the program, inpatient unit staffing patterns, and the initial stages of grant writing and funding.

IMPLEMENTATION OF THE HOSPICE CARE PROGRAM

At this point in the project, the totally developed plan was approved by administration and returned to the board. The plan was submitted with a list of implementation steps to be carried out over a seven-month period. This month-by-month action plan began in July 1982 with the submission of three grant proposals for funds to cover start-up costs and extended through January 1983 with the planned admission of our first patient into the home care program.

Interim steps included the submission of a formal proposal to Blue Cross of Maryland for reimbursement approval, development of orientation materials for staff members, recruitment and selection of team members, contractual arrangements for ambulance services and durable medical supplies, physical renovations of the inpatient unit, and recruitment and training of volunteers.

Of all the planning tools that we used, this month-by-month plan was the most effective. In reflecting back on it, we recognize that some elements were unrealistic, but the end result was that we were able to admit our first home care patient on March 7, 1983, just two months after our target date.

The hiring of staff took place in a planned order. The first position filled was that of the director of hospice care, followed by the coordinator of volunteers, home care coordinator, and inpatient coordinator. The inpatient coordinator then began hiring and training her staff according to patterns that had received prior approval. At the same time, the home care coordinator finalized policies, developed a patient record system, and prepared for certification.

During this implementation phase, the 13-bed inpatient unit was renovated. Staff members who had been involved in the renovation plans emphasized the need for a large family room containing a refrigerator, microwave oven, and table and chairs for eating, as well as comfortable living room furniture; a small quiet room where a patient's relatives and friends could go for privacy or solitude; a whirlpool tub; and a homelike atmosphere throughout the unit. The quiet room contained a foldup cot for the use of visitors who wished to stay overnight with a dying loved one.

It was decided that the hospice would begin providing home care services before the inpatient unit was ready to open. This emphasized the primacy of home care to hospice. The inpatient unit was considered as a backup for short-term admissions, primarily for symptom control and respite care. We did encounter one difficult situation during the period before the inpatient unit opened: a family was unable to manage the patient at home, even with supportive services, and the patient was admitted to the hospital, where he died, just hours before our unit was opened. This was painful to our staff, but in some ways it helped us realize the value of our program with its dual components.

Staffing Patterns: Inpatient Unit

Two inpatient teams were set up, one for six beds and one for seven. This enabled us to hire the first team as we gradually phased in the first seven beds, with plans for bringing the second team on later. The staffing for each six or seven beds is as follows: 7:00–3:00 and 3:00–11:00 shifts: one registered nurse, one nursing technician (a nursing assistant with at least two years' experience at our facility who has passed both written and clinical tests demonstrating advanced knowledge and skills as an assistant), and a nursing assistant. The 11:00-7:00 shift has a registered nurse and a nursing assistant per team, and a nursing technician shared between the two teams. Although we began by staffing one team, we brought two registered nurses on the day shift from the beginning, since the inpatient coordinator had initial organizational responsibilities.

By simple calculation one can determine that this staffing pattern provides 10 or 11 hours of care per patient per day, based on either six or seven beds. Our experience has been that this is not at all excessive. The patients who come to our unit need extensive nursing care in addition to emotional and psychological support. At times we have had to increase the number of volunteers to ensure that dying patients would have someone with them when they expressed a fear of being alone.

Volunteer Component

We were extremely fortunate to be able to hire a master's-prepared social worker with a background in hospice volunteer training. She worked part-time as the hospice care social worker and part-time as the coordinator of volunteers. The other piece of good fortune we experienced was that the Maryland Catholic Health Care Consortium, a coalition of eight Catholic hospitals and nursing homes in the Archdiocese of Baltimore, developed a hospice volunteer training program and tested it in two separate pilot training programs. Since that time, three of the member facilities, including ourselves, have collaborated in offering training programs for hospice volunteers. This has reduced staff time needed for training and has also ensured that the curriculum remains consistent, although the different institutions have varied the length of the training program.

We have slowly but consistently increased the number of volunteers in our program. Initially, we were concerned that we would train too many volunteers before the program needed them: we worried that they might lose interest before being called to duty. Fifteen months after the opening of our home care program, we have 59 trained active volunteers, who serve in home care, the inpatient unit, or both. This number increases with every training session. We have added two follow-up volunteer training days, one for those interested in learning basic nursing-assistant skills, such as how to make a bed or give a bath, and the second in bereavement follow-up. Our bereavement program is run almost exclusively by volunteers and could not exist without them.

Our long-term-care facility had a large volunteer program before the hospice care program began. We considered having only one volunteer program for Stella Maris that would include both long-term care and hospice, but because of the differences between the two types of service and the amount of training required for hospice care, we decided on two separate programs with separate coordinators. After 16 months' experience, I feel that this decision was a wise one and that the programs should continue functioning as established. Our hospice care program would not be what it is without these dedicated, dependable volunteers who have served so freely in our inpatient unit as well as in the home setting.

Reimbursement Issues

I would like to offer some reflections about the reimbursement issue, since it is crucial to survival, and particularly about the new Medicare hospice benefit. Our program was approved by Blue Cross of Maryland as part of its hospice pilot program early in our operations. Our home care services received Medicare approval and our inpatient beds are certified for skilled nursing care under Medicare. We encountered problems in the home care component in obtaining reimbursement for patients who needed hospice home care services but whose medical condition did not correspond to Medicare's skilled-care category. The Medicare reimbursement rate for inpatient services was slightly less than half of the actual costs of hospice inpatient care.

Because of the problems with the traditional Medicare benefit and because our program as it had been designed met the requirements of the Medicare hospice regulations, we began to consider the advantages and disadvantages of seeking certification for this new program. However, the rates set by Medicare for the new program raised as many serious concerns as the traditional Medicare benefit. Would we be able to comply with the 80-20 ratio of home care days to inpatient days? Would the $6,500 cap cause us serious financial hardship? What changes would we have to make if we participated in the program and it was discontinued through the sunset provision in 1986? Perhaps the most serious problems we attempted to anticipate were related to the financial impact of extended hospitalization of a Medicare hospice patient, or several patients who lived beyond the benefit period.

With just six months of experience as a hospice program, we could not adequately answer these questions. We also considered our mission statement in the light of the benefit to the patient and realized the service that this certification could provide to the Medicare-eligible patient. Therefore, with board approval, we applied for and obtained certification as a Medicare hospice provider. Our program has grown steadily since we received this certification. We monitor the admission process closely and have further refined our screening procedures. We are constantly seeking to improve patient and family understanding of the waiving of traditional Medicare benefits if hospice care is elected.

State medical assistance reimbursement (Medicaid) for home care services covers total costs of care if skilled nursing care is needed. However, inpatient reimbursement through Medicaid is very inadequate: it presently covers about 35-45 percent of hospice costs, because we are reimbursed at long-term-care-facility rates, rather than for the level of care that we are actually providing.

We constantly work with businesses and insurance companies to receive approval of our program and reimbursement for services to their clients and employees. Many insurance plans offer a hospice home care benefit but no inpatient coverage. Others, such as Blue Cross, limit the number of inpatient days allowed. It is only on rare occasions that this limitation creates a problem, because hospice care is primarily home care.

We developed a hospice care fund to assist us with the initial costs of operation. Many memorial donations are left as contributions to this fund, and we currently use this money to help finance the care of patients without insurance or a hospice benefit. We have made great strides in obtaining insurance coverage for our patients and program, but it is an unending challenge that requires time, effort, and personal contacts.

ISSUES AFTER ONE YEAR OF OPERATION

There are so many strengths to our long-term-care–based hospice program that it is gratifying to observe its functioning after a year of operation. These strengths include, but are not limited to, the following: quality of staff, working philosophy and team concept, excellent volunteer training and volunteer services, patient and family satisfaction, and staff support groups. Team conferences are held weekly; thus both home care and inpatient staffs are kept aware of the condition of each patient. Transfers between the dual components have worked smoothly and efficiently. Families have commented on the feelings of support and security they have when they bring their loved one to the inpatient unit and are accompanied or greeted by their home care nurse.

A definite strength of our program was the choice of a registered nurse as director. Her nursing knowledge and background have contributed to all aspects of the program. I could elaborate on these strengths indefinitely, but rather, I choose to sum up this paper by saying that what was once a vision has become a vital reality because of the caring, dedication, and professional skills of all members of the hospice team, from the housekeepers and volunteers to the physician.

Needless to say, every program has its problems and concerns, and hospice care is no different. Reimbursement issues are a continual challenge, and we continue to seek cost reimbursement from all providers, including Medicaid and other insurance companies without a hospice benefit or inpatient coverage. The provisions of the Medicare hospice benefit, especially the 80–20 ratio, \$6,500 cap, and waiver of traditional benefits, require constant monitoring. Other concerns from the administrative perspective include the continual fluctuations in patient census, which cause emotional stress on the staff and fiscal strains on the institution. Our budgeting process has been adjusted to address the financial impact of hospice care, and staff support sessions with an outside facilitator attempt to provide staff members with opportunities to express their feelings and concerns.

The nature of hospice care creates an overwhelming need for bereavement services. This has been one of our greatest challenges in our first year of operation. Volunteers with special training have been invaluable in providing this service. We have just approved a part-time position for a bereavement coordinator to oversee this program and coordinate the group sessions.

Other ongoing concerns and challenges include how to provide services to patients who do not have primary caregivers, screening for true hospice patients, and continued education about and marketing of the hospice care concept. We continually try to educate patients, families, and physicians on the differences between our long-term-care beds and the hospice short-term inpatient unit.

As the hospice care program continues to become stable and to grow, our efforts will center on continued marketing and education for the public. Within the institution, we are continally striving to develop a sharing relationship between the long-term-care staff and the hospice staff.

A long-term-care facility provides an excellent base for a hospice care program, but a great deal of planning and background work is necessary to implement such a program.